A – Z
POCKETBOOK
OF
SYMPTOM
CONTROL

by

Peter Kaye
MA MB FRCP MRCGP

CONTENTS

2

CONTENTS

PREFACE

This book is intended for:

- Palliative Care professionals
- General Practitioners
- Junior hospital doctors
- Ward sisters

This book is about controlling symptoms in cancer, (although the same principles apply to many other conditions). It aims to provide an easy-to-use checklist of treatment options. It is meant to be a resource, an aide memoire, and a note-book, but is NOT intended to be a complete statement of management for any particular problem.

Each section provides a simple list of the treatment and management options for a particular problem or symptom. It is not possible to give a definitive order that things should be done (1, 2, 3 then 4), because clinical situations are too complicated and individual. However, I have tried to put the treatment options in the order in which they might usually be considered.

Symptom control is important at each stage of care. The words "palliative", "hospice" and "terminal" imply different stages of illness and different goals:

TYPE OF CARE	PROGNOSIS	FOCUS
Palliative treatment	Months/Years	Prolonging life
Palliative care/ Hospice care	Weeks/Months	Symptom control and quality of remaining life
Terminal care	Days	Patient's comfort and anticipatory grieving of family

The same principles of care apply at each stage, and a multi-disciplinary team of professionals is needed to meet the complex and changing needs of patients and families. The various elements of care (symptom control, rehabilitation, physiotherapy and massage, occupational therapy, social support, expert nursing, counselling, family support, spiritual awareness, terminal care and bereavement follow-up) need to be available wherever the patient is cared for:

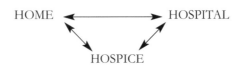

HOME ⟷ HOSPITAL

HOSPICE

This new edition has been completely revised and extensively rewritten, with new sections added on Assessment, Equi-Analgesic Doses, Complementary Therapies, Denial, Emotional Distress, Family Meetings, Drawing a Family Tree, Fentanyl, Itch, Listening Skills, Spiritual Distress, Wound Healing and Patient Information.

The patient information sections about breathlessness and pain can be photocopied and given to patients.

Symptom control is the foundation of good palliative and hospice care, but it is only the first step. The aim of symptom control is to release patients from physical distress so that they can focus on more important issues, such as:

- Rehabilitation
- Changes in role
- Emotional adjustment
- Focus on relationships
- Unfinished business
- Meaning of life

The quality of care we offer depends on the quality of the questions we ask (see Questions).

The principles of symptom control are straightforward, but clinical decision-making can still be very complex. Physical, social, emotional and spiritual dilemmas are often all mixed together. It can take time and sensitivity to clarify the ethically correct course of action. "Writing prescriptions is easy, understanding people is hard" (see Ethical problems).

Explanation is an essential (and greatly neglected) part of symptom control. At one time explanation was all that a physician could usefully offer – and it remains extremely important. Explanation involves teaching. It sometimes has to be done very sensitively (see Breaking Bad News).

Abbreviations have been used to keep the book brief (eg RT for radiotherapy), and are explained in the index.

I am very grateful to Clive Peedell for the sections on chemotherapy, radiotherapy and hormone therapy. I am also very grateful to Anna Spathis, Tabitha Thomas, David Smart, and John Chambers for their helpful comments.

Peter Kaye
Northampton

PRINCIPLES OF SYMPTOM CONTROL

- Listen to the details.
- Ask about ALL symptoms (see list opposite).
- Detailed drug history.
- Ask WHY? Why is the symptom occuring – look for reversible factors.
- Interlace questions about physical symptoms with questions about feelings – this greatly increases the effectiveness of the consultation and the quality of the information (see Questions).
- Treat promptly – symptoms have no more diagnostic usefulness in a situation of advanced disease.
- Make one change at a time (as far as possible).
- Explain changes.
- Include patient in decision-making.
- Involve the relatives.
- Skilful prescribing (see Prescribing).
- Use a drug card.
- Make a plan (eg "What if he vomits").
- Monitor regularly (until symptom-free).
- Remember emotional factors.
- Reduce or stop drugs whenever possible.

NOTES:

The most difficult symptoms to manage in the home are (ABCD):

- Anxiety (if severe)
- Bleeding (if frightening)
- Confusion
- Diarrhoea (if patient is bedbound)

COMMON SYMPTOMS IN ADVANCED CANCER

Weakness	95%
Pain	80%
Anorexia	80%
Constipation	65%
Dyspnoea	60%
Insomnia	60%
Sweats	60%
Oedema	60%
Dry/Sore Mouth	50%
Nausea	50%
Vomiting	40%
Anxiety	40%
Cough	30%
Confusion	30%
Pressure Sore	30%
Pleural effusion	20%
Ascites	15%
Bleeding	15%
Depression	10%
Drowsiness	10%
Itch	5%
Diarrhoea	5%
Fistula	1%

The list above was derived from several surveys, and it is only intended to be a rough guide.

TERMINAL SYMPTOMS
(last 48 hours)

Moist breathing	56%
Pain	51%
Agitation	42%
Incontinence of urine	32%
Dyspnoea	22%
Retention	21%
Nausea and Vomiting	14%
Sweating	14%
Jerking, twitching	12%
Plucking	9%
Confusion	9%

The list above is from a study of 200 <u>hospice</u> patients.
(Lichter and Hunt, J Pall Care 1990; 6: 7–15).

ASSESSMENT

Prepare
- Read the notes
- Are you the right person?
- Talk with relevant others
- SET TIME ASIDE (switch off bleep!)

Introduce yourself
- Smile!
- Give your name and role
- Ask permission to sit down
- Make brief social contact
- Explain the purpose of your visit
- Set a time boundary

Is this the right time?
- Is the patient feeling tired, sick or in pain?
- Is there privacy?
- Have they just been assessed by someone else?
- Do they want anyone else with them?

Start by listening
- Ask "How did the illness start?"
- Ask: "What happened next?"
- Listen to their story
- Understand their perspective\priorities

Formal history – fact finding
- Present illness
- Past Medical History
- Drugs in detail\Allergies
- Symptoms – use a checklist (see previous page)
           – use a body chart to map pains

Identify the main concerns
- Ask "What are your main concerns at the moment?"
- NB This is a very important task of the assessment

Use the technique of interlacing
- Interlace questions about facts with questions about feelings, eg "How did that make you feel?"
- Interlacing increases both patient and professional satisfaction with consultations.

Examine
- Be careful and gentle – do not cause pain, which reduces trust
- It can sometimes be helpful to watch the patient walking
- Take the opportunity to find something to be positive about, eg "Your lungs sound healthy", or "Your joints move well".

Summarize
- Summarizing is a key skill
  eg, "so the main problems are ... and you feel ... is that correct?"
- It clarifies mutual understanding

Draw a family tree (see next page)
- A family tree provides very useful information
- It demonstrates interest in the family
- It builds trust and empathy

Explore psycho-social aspects
- Mobility, Self care, activites of daily living
- Home, job, dependents, pets, responsibilities, hobbies, interests, friends, social activities, religious faith?
- Any other ongoing problems?

Main aim at the moment?
- Ask: "What is your main aim at the moment?"
- A very useful question, that reduces the risk of making incorrect assumptions

Write a drug card
- Essential for good symptom control
- Who is in charge of the medication?
- For inpatients discuss the drug chart with the patient

Explain
- Offer explanations (eg "Is there anything you would like me to explain?"
- Use simple clear language, repeat, use diagrams

Make a plan
- Explore "what if" scenarios, eg "What if I vomit and can't take my tablets?"
- Share decision-making
- The plan should be transferable to different settings
- Arrange follow up

NOTES:

Future care takes less time if there has been a careful first assessment because trust has been established. Questions can be asked at a first assessment that are more difficult to ask later.

Encourage the patient to tell their story. Eg "How did this illness start?" or "I have read through your medical notes but it would help me to know how you yourself see things at the moment". Then listen! Active listening enables you to "tune in" to the patient, and gives you a better understanding of how to talk with the patient.

A family-centred approach increases trust and reduces anxieties (see Family Meetings).

Avoid making assumptions (all patients are different) – ask questions!

Explanations should be written in the notes – it destroys trust when members of the same team give differing explanations.

> *"…if the doctor shows genuine feeling and deep concern for us, and if he or she smiles, then we feel OK. But if the doctor shows little human affection, then even though he or she may be a very great expert, we may feel unsure and nervous. This is human nature"*
>
> *the Dalai Lama*

DRAWING A FAMILY TREE

EXAMPLE OF A FAMILY TREE

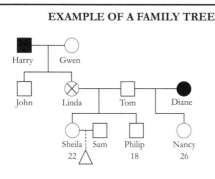

A family tree often highlights important decisions:

- Father, Harry, died of cancer (Does it "run in the family"?)
- Mother, Gwen, is frail ("Should we tell her?")
- Brother, John, lives abroad ("When should he come home?")
- Husband's first wife, Diane, died of cancer "in terrible pain" (explore what happened)
- First grandchild expected in four months ("Will I live to see it born?")
- Son, Philip, is "never at home these days". (Is he too distressed to visit?)
- Step-daughter, Nancy, is estranged. (Should contact be re-established?)

KEY FOR DRAWING A FAMILY TREE

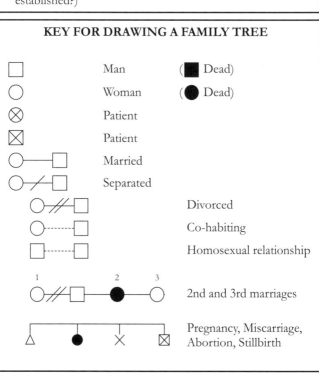

DRAWING A FAMILY TREE

The family tree is a simple and useful communication tool.

Drawing the family tree (or 'genogram') should be a routine part of the assessment of every new patient. It can be drawn by any team member, and can be updated by others as the team meets more of the family. It takes 5–10 minutes and will certainly save time later, because as time goes on it usually becomes increasingly important to know something about the family. It normally incorporates the generations above and below the patient (parents and children). At a glance the structure of the family can be seen, names can be remembered, and new information can be added later. It focuses attention on the family as the unit of care, and reminds the patient of the family support available. It provides a useful record of the family in the clinical notes.

Ask the patient "It would be helpful for us to know a bit more about your family, may I ask you some questions about your family?" The best time is usually at the end of the history, after asking about their main concerns at the moment, and just before the examination. The few minutes spent discussing the family often transforms the consultation. The patient appreciates that you want to be aware of their wider perspective and often feels more relaxed and trustful.

Relevant information often emerges about family relationships and family decisions that can affect clinical management decisions – eg timing of admissions or procedures, and it allows the patient to ask further important questions, eg about genetics.

Most patients have concerns about their family (who have concerns about them) and most feel relieved to know that the professional team has some interest in knowing about who is in their family. Occasionally patients wonder why you want to ask about the family. Explain that an illness in a family usually affects everyone in the family in different ways (which may be a new insight for them) and that it is helpful for the professional team to know who is part of the family.

Family meetings are an important aspect of palliative care, and a family tree is always very helpful when a family meeting is held (see Family Meetings).

30 KEY SKILLS FOR PALLIATIVE CARE

Skill 1: Active listening

Skill 2: Giving clear explanations

Skill 3: Breaking bad news whilst maintaining hope

Skill 4: Gaining the trust of a patient

Skill 5: Assessing a patient's needs

Skill 6: Taking a drug history

Skill 7: Managing a patient in denial

Skill 8: Working alongside sadness

Skill 9: Drawing a family tree

Skill 10: Talking to relatives

Skill 11: Helping a patient to control visitors

Skill 12: Dealing with your own feelings

Skill 13: Discussing sexual problems

Skill 14: Recognising spiritual distress

Skill 15: Applying the principles of symptom control

Skill 16: Applying drug pharmacology

Skill 17: Managing cancer pain

Skill 18: Managing nausea and vomiting

Skill 19: Preventing constipation

Skill 20: Using a syringe driver

Skill 21: Using a drug card

Skill 22: Using morphine

Skill 23: Using fentanyl

Skill 24: Understanding equi-analgesic doses

Skill 25: Managing insomnia

Skill 26: Managing panic attacks

Skill 27: Managing spinal cord compression

Skill 28: Recognising dying

Skill 29: Visiting a dying patient

Skill 30: Supporting a bereaved family

NOTES:

Use this tick-box list to check your own expertise and to monitor your own abilities or learning needs.

More experienced practitioners can use this as a teaching list – Which areas am I competent to teach? Which do I need to review?

Skills depend on 3 things:

1. **Beliefs**. Having the right underlying attitudes, eg no patient should have to put up with pain.

2. **Knowledge**. Having the correct level of knowledge, which is derived from teaching, reading, observing and reflecting on your own experience, preferably with others.

3. **Motivation**. Having the willingness and energy to use the skills. Knowing how to do something well does not mean you <u>will</u> do it well.

ANALGESICS 1 – Weak Opioids

NON-OPIOIDS

- Paracetamol 1g QID
- NSAIDs (See NSAIDs)

WEAK OPIOIDS

- Codeine 60mg 4 hourly
- Dihydrocodeine 60mg 4 hourly
- DHC Continus 60–120mg 12 hourly
- Co-proxamol 2 tablets QID
- Tramadol 50–100mg QID

Paracetamol 1g QID can control mild cancer pains and is the first step on the analgesic ladder. It will also control some pains that are unrelieved by morphine, eg tension headache. It acts centrally, inhibiting the production of prostaglandins in the brain. It is hepatotoxic in overdose. Safe with alcohol.

Codeine 30–60 mg 4 hourly is used for moderate pain. It is very constipating. It is methyl-morphine and is metabolized to morphine and mainly acts as a pro-drug of morphine, but 1/10 as potent. It is often used in compound analgesics, eg co-codamol (see table below).

Dihydrocodeine 30–60mg 4 hourly is equipotent to codeine. It is a semi-synthetic analogue of codeine.

DHC Continus tablets M\R. 60mg 90mg 120mg contain dihydrcodeine in slow release form. It is effective BD, and useful to reduce the number of tablets needed.

Co-proxamol contains 32.5mg dextropropoxyphene, a synthetic derivative of methadone. It is a weak mu agonist, equipotent with codeine. It causes less nausea, drowsiness and dry mouth than low dose morphine. Also acts at NMDA receptor as mild antagonist (? clinically relevant).

ANALGESICS 1 – Weak Opioids

Tramadol (Zydol) 50–100mg QID is an effective medium strength analgesic. It is a "dual action" analgesic. It increases spinal levels of noradrenaline and 5HT (by blocking their re-uptake) which activates the inhibitory pain fibres that travel down from the midbrain. It is also a mild mu agonist, and can cause constipation. It is rapidly absorbed. Analgesia begins within 1 hour and peaks within 2 hours. It is less effective than morphine for severe pain, but can be equivalent to morphine for moderate pain. It causes fewer side effects than morphine. It can cause hypotension. There is a theoretical risk of fits if given with tricyclics or SSRIs.

COMPOUND ANALGESICS

	WEAK OPIOID		+	NON-OPIOID	
CO-PROXAMOL	= dextropropoxyphene	32.5mg	+	paracetamol	325mg
CO-CODAMOL	= codeine	30mg	+	paracetamol	500mg
CO-DYDRAMOL	= dihydrocodeine	10mg	+	paracetamol	500mg
CO-CODAPRIN	= codeine	8mg	+	aspirin	400mg

Notes:

Non opioids and opioids should be used together before considering the co-analgesics (see Pain 3).

ANALGESICS 2 – Strong Opioids

Morphine – Still the gold standard (see Morphine)

Diamorphine
- Used for injections and infusions
- 15 × more soluble than morphine (120mg dissolves in 0.2ml water).
- Conversion ratio 3:1 with oral morphine (some use 2:1)
- Monitor carefully after conversion (?pain, ?drowsy)
- For dose conversions see Analgesics 3

Fentanyl (see Fentanyl)	• Transdermal patch lasts 3 days • Actiq lozenges ('lollipops') short-acting

Oxycodone

Oxynorm (4 hourly)
5mg – orange/beige
10mg – white/beige
20mg – pink/beige
Liquid 1mg/5ml,
  10mg/1ml

Oxycontin (12 hourly)
5mg – blue
10mg – white
20mg – pink
40mg – yellow

- Semi-synthetic opioid
- Similar to morphine (more active at kappa)
- Possibly less nausea and confusion than morphine
- Twice as potent as morphine (5mg to 10mg morphine)
- Safe in renal failure
- About 5% of the white population are 'slow metabolisers' of oxycodone and may need lower doses

Hydromorphone

Palladone (4 hourly)
1.3mg – orange/clear
2.6mg – red/clear

Palladone SR (12 hourly)
2mg – yellow/clear
4mg – light blue/clear
8mg – pink/clear
16mg – brown/clear
24mg – dark blue/clear

- Acts at mu receptors like morphine
- No advantages over oxycodone
- 8 × more potent than morphine (1.3 mg to 10mg morphine)
- safe in renal failure
- May cause fewer side effects than morphine

Methadone
- Synthetic opioid
- Mu and delta agonist and NMDA-receptor antagonist
- Well absorbed from all routes (orally, rectally or by injection)
- Half-life up to 80 hours, it accumulates and repeated doses can cause drowsiness, even after several days at a steady dose. Monitor carefully.
- Fewer side-effects than morphine
- Difficult to convert from morphine to methadone – usually requires period as an inpatient. The usual loading dose is a tenth of the 24 hour morphine dose, e.g. if the patient is on 300mg\24h of oral morphine, give 30mg methadone stat then 15mg BD, with 15mg for breakthrough pain.
- The final dose of methadone is usually in the range of 10–40mg BD, which is usually around one tenth the previous 24 hour dose of oral morphine.
- Since it differs from morphine, a simple and logical way of using it is to simply add a low static dose, such as 10mg BD, to the present morphine regime, for its NMDA effect, eg for neuropathic pain.
- Safe in renal failure (no active metabolites)
- SCI possible (use half 24h oral dose) but causes inflammation
- Interacts with phenytoin and carbamazepine (decreased methadone levels) and with fluconazole and SSRIs (which increase methadone levels).

NOTES:

Fears of addiction or respiratory depression are unfounded (see Pain 4). Opioids can be reversed with naloxone or naltroxone – rarely needed.

Analgesics 3 – Equi-analgesic doses

CONVERSION TABLE FOR <u>ORAL</u> ANALGESICS

ANALGESIC	ORAL DOSE	ORAL MORPHINE EQUIVALENT (4 hourly)
WEAK OPIOIDS		
Codeine	60mg	5mg
Dihydrocodeine	60mg	5mg
Co-proxamol	2 tabs	5mg
Tramadol	50mg	5mg
Pethidine (oral)*	50mg	5mg
Pentazocine*	50mg	5mg
STRONG OPIOIDS		
Oxycodone	5mg	10mg
Hydromorphone	1.3mg	10mg
Dipipanone* (in Diconal)	1 tab	10mg
Buprenorphine* tablet	0.2mg	10mg
Meptazinol*	200mg	10mg
Dextromoramide	5mg	15mg
Actiq lozenge (buccal)	200mcg	5mg
Methadone	5mg	5–25mg
PATCHES		
Fentanyl (Durogesic)	25 mcg\hr	15mg
Buprenorphine* (Transtec)	35 mcg\hr	5mg

* Not recommended for Palliative Care

CONVERTING TO DIAMORPHINE

24hr MORPHINE (oral)	24hr DIAMORPHINE (SC infusion)	PRN DIAMORPHINE (single SC injection) For breakthrough pain
60mg (10mg 4 hourly)	20mg	2.5mg
90mg (15mg 4 hourly)	30mg	5mg

NOTES:

The main reasons for changing a strong opioid ("opioid rotation") are either side effects or poor pain control. *Clinically* the opioids are very similar in terms of analgesia and side-effects, and changing from one to another is unlikely to make a profound difference. *Pharmacologically* we still know very little about how the strong opioids differ from each other. Look for other causes of side effects (nausea, confusion) or poor pain control BEFORE changing opioid.

The table opposite provides all the information needed to safely convert from one strong oral opioid to another. Use oral morphine dosage as a common "currency" when converting from one opioid to another. Using the correct conversion ratio, you can be confident that you will be giving the patient a safe dose of the new analgesic that will control their pain without causing severe side effects.

Conversion to a different opioid happens in two stages:

1) Calculate the correct equi-analgesic dose range (see table)

2) Monitor carefully over the first day and *fine-tune* the dose for that patient; if pain breakthrough increase the dose a bit, if painfree but a bit drowsy, reduce the dose a bit.

Methadone is different to the other strong opioids because of its very long half-life. A single dose is approximately equi-analgesic to morphine, but with repeated dosing it accumulates and becomes stronger. (See Analgesics 2)

See Also: Fentanyl.

ANOREXIA

Exclude Reversible Causes	• Anxiety or Depression • Nausea • Thrush • Constipation • Drugs (digoxin, cytotoxics)
Dexamethasone 2–4mg\day	• Helps 80% • Effect may only last 1–2 weeks • Side-effects can be a problem • See Steroids
Metoclopramide (Maxolon) 10–20g TID	• Before meals • Reduces fullness\heartburn of gastric stasis.
Progestagen	• eg medroxyprogesterone (Provera) 100–200mg daily • Optimum dose unknown • Improves appetite • Mode of action unknown • Alternative to steroids if prognosis is still in months • Improvement may take 1–2 weeks
Multivitamins	• Can help 40–50% (Placebo effect)
Refer to dietitian?	• Dietary needs • Feeding proplems • Wide range of supplements • Psychologically very important for some patients.
Try new foods\tastes	• 20% have taste changes • Preferences often change • Herbs and spices can help
Food Presentation	• Small portions • Attractive presentation helps • Eat little and often • Microwave helps to prepare meals as needed
Educate family	• Eating can be tiring • High food intake does not improve prognosis. • Tastes can change. • Use of convenience foods • Sedentary life-style only needs 1500 calories per day. • Dietary advice can help (refer to a dietitian).

Nutritional Supplements	• eg Ensure, Fresubin, Fortisip • Wide range of flavours • Nutritionally complete (energy, protein, fat, vitamins) • Sip feeding (50–100ml per hr) • Usually 200–400cc\day • 2L\day provide full nutrition (eg via gastrostomy)
Advice	• Maintain fluid intake • No foods are harmful • Eat when hungry • Avoid regular weighing (demoralizing)

NOTES:

Taste changes are common in advanced cancer (20%). They include sudden dislikes, new preferences, or foods may taste "strange". A metallic taste may follow chemotherapy. Extra seasoning of food (herbs and spices) can help. Add salt if too sweet, or sugar if too bitter. Taste changes are not necessarily permanent, and after several weeks taste can return to normal. Zinc deficiency has been implicated as a cause. A bad taste in the mouth suggests thrush, gingivitis or bleeding.

Intensive feeding (NG or IV) does not improve appetite, weight, well-being or prognosis in advanced cancer and has no place in the management of anorexia. Gastrostomy has a place in the management of dysphagia (see Gastrostomy).

ANTI-EMETICS

1ST LINE ANTI-EMETICS

Metoclopramide
PO: 10–20mg QID
SCI: 30–100mg\24h
SC,IM: 10mg

- Used in 75% of prescriptions for N&V
- Especially for large volume vomiting due to gastric stasis, because it is gastro-kinetic.
- Also has a central action
- Can cause dystonic side-effects

Haloperidol
PO: 1.5–3mg OD
SCI: 2.5–10mg\24h
SC: 2.5mg

- Used in 50% of prescriptions for N&V
- Especially for chemical causes (when nausea is often more pronounced than vomiting)
- Can cause dystonic side-effects

Cyclizine
PO: 50mg TID
SCI: 150mg\24h
IM: 50mg

- For bowel obstruction, movement-related nausea or raised ICP (with steroids).
- Acts on both histamine and cholinergic receptors in the vomiting centre.
- Has anti-cholinergic side-effects
- Can be effectively combined with haloperidol

2ND LINE ANTI-EMETICS

Levomepromazine
PO: 6.25mg OD
SCI: 12.5 mg\24h

- Broad-spectrum anti-emetic
- Can be effective when first line drugs have failed
- Drowsiness

Dexamethasone
PO: 4–8mg OD
SCI: 4–12mg\24h
IM: 4–8mg OD

- Effective add-on – increases the effect of other drugs
- Used for both chemically-induced vomiting and bowel obstruction
- May reduce permeability of CTZ to emetogenic chemicals, but mode of action is not fully understood

Granisetron
PO: 1–2mg BD
SCI: 1–2mg

- Very effective for post-chemotherapy vomiting
- Synergistic with haloperidol
- Effective in uraemia and bowel obstruction (because 5HT is released from the inflamed gut and from platelets damaged by uraemia).

NOTES:

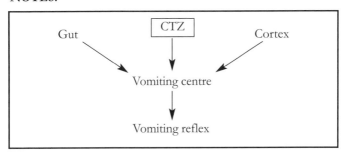

It is logical to combine anti-emetics that act at different receptors, eg cyclizine with haloperidol. Note that levomepromazine is a broad-spectrum anti-emetic that acts at several different receptors.

RECEPTOR BLOCKADE BY ANTI-EMETICS						
	CTZ		Vomiting Centre		Gut Wall	
RECEPTORS:	D2	5HT2	H1	Cholin	5HT3	5HT4
Metoclopramide	++				+	++
Haloperidol	+++					
Cyclizine			++	++		
Levomepromazine	++	+++	+++	++		
Granisetron					+++	
Hyoscine hydrobromide			+++			

The chemo-receptor trigger zone (CTZ) has dopamine type 2 receptors (D2) stimulated by drugs (eg opioids) and by chemicals in the blood (urea, calcium). It also has 5–HT2 receptors, blocked by levomepromazine, and cannabinoid receptors.

The vomiting centre has receptors for histamine (H1) and for acetyl choline. It also receives input from the CTZ, gut, cortex, inner ear, intense pain and touch fibres in the throat.

The gut has 5HT3 receptors, found in 1986. They activate the vagus nerves, and are the cause of chemotherapy-induced vomiting.

Pro-kinetic drugs act on 5–HT4 receptors in the gut to increase peristalsis (domperidone and metoclopramide)

The cerebal cortex has benzodiazepine receptors. *Lorazepam* is an effective anti-emetic but is very sedating.

ANXIETY

Assessment	• Is it long-standing?
	• When and where?
	• Specific fears?
	• Total denial?
	• Physical symptoms?
	   – sweats
	   – tremor
	   – palpitations
	• Panic attacks?
	• Poor sleep? Nightmares?
	• Poor concentration?

Lorazepam	• INDICATIONS:
	   • poor sleep
	   • poor concentration
	   • panic attacks
	• 0.5–1mg PRN or TID
	• Useful anxiolytic
	• Half-life 8–25 hours
	• Effective sublingually
	• SEE table opposite

Amitriptyline	• 25–100mg nocte • Agitated depression can mimic anxiety
Olanzepine	• 2.5–10mg OD • Useful for agitation or paranoia • Atypical anti-psychotic • Dopamine antagonist • Fewer side effects than typical ones • Little sedation • Long half-life (34 hours) • Parkinsonism can still occur
Propranolol	• 10–40mg QID • Controls tremor\palpitations of anxiety • Consider excluding thyrotoxicosis • Contra-indicated in asthma
Counselling	• Most anxiety responds to listening and support. • Patients adjust by finding new solutions and new ways of thinking. • Elicit specific fears by asking "What is the worse thing that could happen?". • NB Verbal reassurance is LESS reassuring than listening to feelings and fears
Relaxation Therapy	• Often more effective than anxiolytics • Increases patient's sense of control • Best if teaching session precedes loan of relaxation tapes

Massage	• Relaxes • Physical touch is comforting • Reduces isolation
Family meeting	• Ask patient's permission • Patient anxiety often reflects family anxiety • Patient anxiety may be <u>about</u> family • Reduces sense of isolation • Ask each member "How is the situation affecting <u>your</u> life"? • Families that are brought together will talk together.
Cognitive Psychotherapy	• Helps patient understand how thoughts affect feelings • Indicated especially for patients who have lost control of feelings (eg constant fear) • Refer to psychologist?

ORAL ANXIOLYTICS

		Starting Dose		HALF-LIFE (HOURS) Average	Range
buspirone	(Buspar)	5–10mg	TID	7	2–11
lorazepam	(Ativan)	1–2mg	BD	12	8–25
chlordiazepoxide	(Librium)	10mg	TID	12	6–15
alprazolam	(Xanox)	0.25mg	BD	14	6–20
clobazam	(Frisium)	10mg	TID	18	9–30
diazepam	(Valium)	5mg	OD	32	21–46

NOTES:

Longstanding anxiety may be impossible to change – set realistic goals for management.

Denial is a common cause of anxiety. Avoid giving unrequested information, which increases anxiety. Patient's move towards acceptance at their own rate, helped by feeling secure, and by having professional carers who are trusted, and who offer opportunities for talking about feelings (see Denial).

Extreme anxiety can mimic confusion.

Midazolam can be added to an SC infusion to control anxiety, starting dose 10mg per 24 hours.

ASCITES

Assessment	• Distension • Shifting dullness (detects 500ml) • Ultrasound scan (detects 100ml)
Chemotherapy	• Usually if prognosis is in months • Can resolve ascites due to carcinoma of the breast or ovary.
Peritoneo-venous Shunt	• eg Denver shunt • Simple procedure • Indicated for recurrent ascites in a relatively fit patient. • 30% occlude after 3–6 months and need replacing.
Paracentesis	• Simple drainage procedure • Drain 5–10 litres over 1–3 hours • Slower drainage if frail (hypotension) • Partial drainage if weak\terminal • Diuretics can slow re-accumulation of fluid
Bleomycin	• Intraperitoneal • Slows recurrence of ascites • 90mg in 2 litres instilled then drained off after 15 minutes • IV hydrocortisone 100mg reduces febrile reaction
Spironolactone	• 200–400mg daily reduces ascites over 2–3 weeks • Add frusemide 40–80mg for quicker initial effect • Monitor effect (girth measurements) • Monitor for dehydration (reduce doses)
IV Frusemide	• 100mg\24 hours by slow infusion • Alternative to paracentesis for rapid relief of tense ascites
Morphine	• Controls discomfort\dyspnoea • May be more appropriate than paracentesis if prognosis is in days
PPl	• eg omeprazole 20–40mg OD • Control of reflux oesophagitis • Add metoclopramide 10–20mg QID if severe

NOTES:

Ascites means fluid in the peritoneal cavity. It occurs in cancers of the bronchus and breast due to peritoneal metastases, as well as from intra-abdominal tumours.

Paracentesis is a simple procedure for the rapid relief of tense ascites. The patient should have an empty bladder. The needle is inserted 10 cm away from the midline (to avoid blood vessels) in the left or right iliac fossa. It is contra-indicated if there is intestinal obstruction or multiple adhesions. Vitamin K may be needed first, to reverse warfarin. Paracentesis can safely be repeated, and is usually the best way to control symptomatic ascites in far-advanced disease.

BLEEDING

Radiotherapy	<ul><li>Controls haemoptysis in 90%</li><li>Controls visceral bleeding</li><li>Controls surface bleeding</li></ul>
Tranexanic acid	<ul><li>500mg–1g QID</li><li>Tablets or syrup</li><li>Very effective haemostatic</li><li>May worsen thrombosis</li><li>May worsen bladder clots</li><li>Enema can be made (5g in 50ml water)</li></ul>
Topical Adrenaline	<ul><li>1 in 1000</li><li>Stops capillary bleeding</li><li>Used when dressings changed</li></ul>
Alginate dressing	<ul><li>eg Kaltostat</li><li>Haemostatic dressing</li></ul>
Sucralfate (Antepsin)	<ul><li>2g (10 ml) BD</li><li>Contains aluminium</li><li>Can reduce gastric bleeding</li><li>1g + KY jelly makes a topical paste</li></ul>
1% Alum	<ul><li>Bladder irrigation</li><li>Via 3–way catheter (IL/day)</li><li>Best treatment for bladder haemorrhage</li><li>Alum pack for rectal bleeding</li></ul>
PPl e.g. Omeprazole	<ul><li>For haemorrhagic oesophagitis or gastritis</li></ul>
Laser	<ul><li>Via endoscope</li><li>Lung, stomach, bladder, rectum</li></ul>
Surgical Methods	<ul><li>Nasal pack (ENT Surgeon)</li><li>Diathermy (eg nose)</li><li>Cryotherapy (eg skin)</li><li>Hydrostatic dilation of bladder</li><li>Total cystectomy</li></ul>
Embolization	<ul><li>Especially useful for renal bleeding</li><li>Pelvic bleeding (int. iliac artery)</li><li>Refer to radiologist</li></ul>
Stop Warfarin	<ul><li>Effect wears off over 2–3 days</li><li>IV Vitamin K 1–5mg reverses in several hours</li><li>Fresh frozen plasma is needed to reverse quickly</li></ul>

Platelet Transfusion	•	Effect is short-lived
	•	Considered if marrow failure is causing distressing bleeds (eg retinal, nose)
Blood transfusion	•	Usually only considered once bleeding is controlled – otherwise it worsens bleeding.

NOTES:

Radiotherapy can control bleeding from the lung, oesophagus, rectum, bladder, kidney, uterus or vagina. Surface bleeding from malignant nodes or fungation (cutaneous malignancy) of skin can be controlled, provided there has been no previous radical RT to the area. The perineum or vulva are very sensitive and tolerate RT poorly, and skin reaction can be severe.

Tranexamic acid 500mg–1g QID is a very useful and effective drug to control internal or surface bleeding.

Embolization of bleeding arteries is possible for kidney, lung and sometimes pelvis (internal iliac artery). An interventional radiologist inserts a catheter into the femoral artery under local anaesthetic, and guides the catheter into the relevant arterial system, and injects radio-opaque dye to demonstrate the leaking vessel. The vessel is then embolized with PVA particles or a metal coil, the size depending on the size of the vessel. Large tumours can be embolized in stages.

1% Alum solution must be freshly made up. It controls bleeding by precipitating on the mucosa and constricting capillaries. It is non-toxic. Bladder irrigation with 1l every 12–24 hours can settle bleeding over 1–3 days.

Haematemesis is often due to non-malignant causes in cancer patients, such as peptic ulcer or haemorrhagic oesophagitis due to acid reflux or candida.

Vaginal bleeding is occasionally a problem, eg from hormone therapy. It can be controlled, if necessary, with Norethisterone 5 mg TID or Depo-Provera 50 mg IM.

BREAKING BAD NEWS

1. Convene a meeting	• When? – Soon • Where? – Quiet room with enough chairs • Who? – Ask patient if they want a relative present
2. What does the patient know?	• <u>Narrative of events by patient</u> • eg "Can you help me by telling me what you understand about your illness" or • eg "How did it all start?"
3. What does the patient WANT to know?	• eg "Would you like me to tell you anything else about your illness?" • Acknowledge fear of knowing more • NB Never impose information

4. Narrow the information-gap (?)	• Know all the facts!
	• Start from patient's understanding
	• Use patient's words
	• Warning shot ("There is a tumour")
	• Allow denial
	• <u>Narrative of events by doctor</u> (if wanted)
	   • eg "Would you like me to explain more"
	   • Ask: "Is this making sense?"
	   • NB Avoid medical jargon
	   • NB Avoid too many facts and figures

5. Allow ventilation of feelings (KEY PHASE)	• Acknowledge distress • "How are you feeling now?" • "Is this information a shock?" • Explore concerns • Avoid arguments! • Note – the patient's crisis is NOT your crisis • Listen
6. Make a plan	• Summarize patient's concerns • Discuss future treatment • Be optimistic • Fix date for review
7. Offer to meet family separately	• "Would you like me to talk with anyone else in your family?" • Assess information-gap in same way as above • Give each person an opportunity to speak • Encourage parents to inform children

BREAKING BAD NEWS

NOTES:

Bad news means any information that alters a patient's view of their future for the worse. The way bad news is first imparted can affect both the patient's and the family's ability to cope. The purpose of explaining the situation is to reduce uncertainty about the future, to reduce inappropriate hope (which is demoralizing) to enable appropriate adjustments to be made and to maintain a relationship of trust between patient and professionals. A conspiracy of silence usually causes anxiety or depression ("What is happening to me?") and guilt ("Am I doing something wrong?") and can cheat a person of the opportunity to use his or her remaining time for things that are important.

The meeting: set time aside (diary) arrange for privacy and quiet, avoid interruptions (give your bleep to someone else!) and sit, DON'T stand. It is often best for a doctor and nurse to see the patient and relative(s) together. Make sure there is a close family member present whenever possible. If the patient is alone (which should be avoided) they may be in a state of shock. How will they get home? Who will be at home? NB Avoid giving bad news over the phone – arrange a meeting.

A narrative of event by the patient allows you to find out about the patient's concerns. It is essential that information given <u>matches</u> the information the patient actually wants.

The warning shot: Start by using the patient's word, but find out what they mean by their word (eg "lump"). Titrate new information in a graded way. A *heirarchy of euphemisms* can be useful as a start, (shadow, problem, lump, tumour, cancer) but words may later need to be explained. Allow denial at any stage and do not give unrequested information, which can cause anger\anxiety.

Avoid assumptions eg if a patient asks "How long will it be?" the best reply may be "What have you been thinking?" – it could be that the patient means "how long before I can get back to work?", rather than: "how long before I die?"

Explanation must be clear and simple. Facts and figures will not be remembered and detailed explanations (eg of treatment options) should take place later ("Once he told me I didn't hear anything else"). Avoid jargon, which confuses. Medical words are used to distance the professional from their own emotional distress.

Start with optimism eg "There are things we can do to help, but it is not possible to cure your liver problem". Optimism is supportive, pessimism is not. Avoid harsh statements eg "The cancer is incurable".

Adjustment to bad news, to a different future, takes time and is similar to a process of grief. The person is shocked and needs support and time to adjust. If bad news is explained properly, anxiolytics are rarely needed.

Further reading: *Breaking Bad News – A Ten Step Approach,* by Peter Kaye. E.P.L. Publications. ISBN 0-9519895-7-X.

BREATHLESSNESS 1

Assessment	<ul><li>Severity<ul><li>stairs?</li><li>walking?</li><li>at rest?</li></ul></li><li>Episodic worsening suggests hyperventilation</li><li>Panic attacks?</li><li>Full examination</li><li>Hb\CXR\Peak flow\ECG</li><li>Pulse oximetry (below 90 = hypoxia)</li></ul>
Treat Reversible Causes (*Anaemia is discussed on page 157*)	<ul><li>Tumour mass – RT\chemotherapy</li><li>Anaemia – Transfusion</li><li>Bronchospasm – Bronchodilators</li><li>Heart failure – Diuretics</li><li>Chest infection – Antibiotics</li><li>Pleural effusion – Aspiration</li><li>Pericardial effusion – Pericardiotomy</li><li>Pneumothorax – Chest drain</li><li>Pulmonary emboli – Anti-coagulation</li><li>Arrhythmia – Anti-arrhythmics</li><li>Anxiety – Relaxation</li></ul>
Low-dose morphine	<ul><li>Oramorph 2.5–20mg 4 hourly</li><li>Mechanism unknown</li></ul>
Steroids	<ul><li>Dexamethasone 6–12mg\day</li><li>Useful for lung metastases, lymphangitis, tumour mass or bronchospasm.</li><li>Reduced peri-tumour oedema increases gas exchange</li></ul>
Bronchodilators	<ul><li>Use a spacer device (eg Volumatic) for ordinary inhalers</li><li>Nebulized salbutamol 2.5 or 5mg\2ml PRN or 4 hourly</li><li>Nebulized ipratropium 250–500 mcg\2ml PRN or 4 hourly</li><li>Monitor with peak flow meter</li></ul>
A draft of cold air	<ul><li>eg Electric fan or draught from window</li><li>Proven benefit in breathlessness (Schwartzstein, 1987)</li><li>Needs to be on centre of face</li><li>Try before considering oxygen</li><li>Hand-held battery fan is useful</li><li>Cold water on face can have similar effect</li></ul>
Nebulized saline	<ul><li>Can help, especially if producing sputum</li><li>Nebulized morphine is no more effective</li></ul>

Oxygen	• Reduces dyspnoea at rest from lung tumours, metastases, effusion or lymphangitis. • Use nasal prongs • Use 28% oxygen if chronic bronchitic • Consider pulse oximetry
Lorazepam	• 0.5–1mg PRN or TID • Anxiety and agitation increase oxygen consumption
Relaxation therapy	• Episodes of hyperventilation or panic are a very common feature in most patients with dyspnoea.
Breathing Exercises	• Lower shoulders, breathe right out. • Move abdomen out with inspiration. • Gives patient feeling of control • Refer to physiotherapist
Nursing	• Sit upright\help moving • Table fan • Pillow table • Air blowing onto the face is often comforting. • Quiet room • Companionship • May be easier to nurse in reclining chair (eg Parker Knoll)
Sedation If terminal	• S.C. midazolam plus diamorphine is effective • Necessary for distressing unrelieved or terminal dyspnoea • IV if very distressed • Negotiate carefully with patient!

NOTES:

Breathlessness can be assessed for severity, like pain, by asking the patient to give it a score of 0–10. It is managed differently depending whether it is:

- On exertion   (due to weakness, non-drug methods best)
- At rest   (morphine and oxygen can help)
- Terminal   (may need titrated sedation)

The following are important: *explanation* (eg "an awareness of heavy breathing, like after exercise, can feel unpleasant but is not harmful in itself"), *help in adjusting* to limitations (both physical and psychological), *counselling* to diffuse fears (especially suffocating to death), *a plan of action* for acute episodes at home and *reassurance* that the patient will not be left alone fighting for breath.

BREATHLESSNESS 2

PATIENT INFORMATION

Why do I feel breathless? Disease can make the lungs stiffer and less elastic. This makes it harder to get air down to the air sacs, and sends messages to the brain to breathe harder. Many people with breathlessness have perfectly adequate levels of oxygen in the bloodstream.

Do not get too frightened or upset if you become breathless. Breathlessness is not harmful in itself, even though it can feel very unpleasant. It is important to remain as active as you can.

Normally when we breathe hard, like after running, we breathe faster and our shoulders go up and down. But now, these natural responses tend to aggravate your feelings of breathlessness, because rapid breathing and tense shoulder muscles use more oxygen. It helps to keep your shoulders relaxed and breathe slowly.

Breathing exercises to slow breathing and relax the shoulders can help you cope with feelings of breathlessness. Learn to relax your shoulders down, and do abdominal breathing (singer's breathing) so your abdomen moves out when you breathe in. A physiotherapist can teach you this. Practise this technique a few times during the day.

Breathe in through the nose and out through the mouth. Nose breathing moistens and filters the air before it reaches your lungs.

Plan your activities so that you can do them in small steps. Stop whatever activity is making you breathless, sit down and wait for it to ease off. Do not carry heavy bags, as this can make breathlessness worse. Try to avoid bending over, which can make breathing more difficult.

Relaxation can be very effective in reducing the feeling of breathlessness. Learn some ways of reducing anxiety or panic. Ask your doctor or nurse for a relaxation audiotape. Consider learning how to meditate. As one person with breathlessness said "Now when I feel breathless, I know what to think".

Eating may be difficult due to shortness of breath. Small, frequent meals may be easier than three large meals a day. Nutritional supplements, such as Ensure or Fortisip, can be prescribed by your G.P.

Talking on the phone can be difficult. Get an answer phone or ask friends to let the phone ring for a long time so that you don't have to rush to the phone. Talk in short sentences. Pause after each sentence.

You may need to rest at several points throughout the day. Try to balance periods of rest with some gentle exercise. Do a little at a time so that you don't become exhausted.

Making love is often an area of concern. Talk to your partner about any fears you have. Use positions that minimise breathlessness. Avoid positions that may make you claustrophobic. Try to ensure that you are in a comfortable and well supported position.

Think ahead. Work out tactics for coping with situations which make you panicky. For example being in the bathroom may make you feel claustrophobic, in which case try having the window slightly open.

Try using an electric fan. A draught of air across the face produced by the fan can reduce the feelings of breath-lessness for many people.

Morphine is generally used to treat pain, but a small dose of morphine can be very helpful for reducing the feeling of breathlessness, especially if it is occurring at rest.

Oxygen may help breathlessness *in some people* but it does not help everyone, because oxygen levels are often normal.

A common fear is of dying gasping for breath. In fact it is always possible to control the distress of breathlessness with medication. You will be offered drugs that relax the breathing, and keep you free of the feeling of distress each time you breath. They can make you feel drowsy, but the dose can be balanced to keep you comfortable.

CHEMOTHERAPY (Palliative)

Small cell lung Cancer	<ul><li>With Limited disease (one hemithorax) 90% respond, CR 50%. Median survival 3 months increased to 15 months</li><li>With Extensive Disease 70% respond, CR 25%. Median survival of 6 weeks increased to 8 months</li><li>1st choice is cisplatin plus etoposide, or occasionally CAV (cyclophosphamide, doxorubicin, vincristine)</li><li>2nd line topotecan has 30% response but only 5% CR</li><li>Only 6% survive 2 years, despite high initial response rates</li></ul>
Non-small cell lung cancer	<ul><li>Platinum regimens improve median survival by 2–3 months, for patients with good performance status (0–2)</li><li>1 year survival improved by 10%</li><li>Cisplatin, vinblastine, vinorelbine, mitomycin C, gemcitabine are used</li><li>Docetaxel as a 2nd line</li></ul>
Breast cancer	<ul><li>Good evidence for improved quality of life with chemotherapy</li><li>70% respond (median duration 8–14 months)</li><li>Regular bisphosphonates reduce bone pain and skeletal morbidity</li><li>Chemo is indicated for life threatening visceral involvement (liver/lung mets) even if hormone responsive</li><li>Commonly used combinations include FEC (5–FU, epirubicin, cyclophosphamide), CMF (cyclophosphamide, methotrexate, 5–FU) and MMM (mitomycin C, methotrexate, mitoxantrone)</li><li>2nd line chemo 30% respond (6–12 months), 3rd line 10–25% respond</li><li>Newer agents include vinorelbine, taxotere and paclitaxel</li></ul>
Colorectal cancer	<ul><li>30% response to 5–FU and folinic acid (improve median survival by 6 months)</li><li>Recently, new agents (irinotecan and oxaliplatin) with 5–FU have further improved response rates (to 35–50%) and survival (by a further 2–3 months)</li><li>Oral capecitabine is as effective as IV 5–FU</li></ul>

CHEMOTHERAPY (Palliative)

Gastric and Oesophageal cancer	• Response rates are 40–50% (with median survival 9 months) • ECF (epirubicin, cisplatinum and infusional 5FU) is used for adenocarcinomas. Cisplatin and 5–FU for oesophageal squamous carcinomas
Pancreatic cancer	• Oral gemcitabine is the most active agent • Low response rates, but clinical benefit in 25% and 1 year survival of 18% • No proven benefit for combination chemotherapy
Bladder cancer	• 40–60% respond , 10% CRs • Median survival increased from 3 months to 15 months. • M-VAC (methotrexate, vinblastine, doxorubicin, cisplatin) is used, but is toxic. Alternatively, gemcitabine and cisplatin are less toxic and as effective.
Ovarian cancer	• With advanced disease 65–75% respond, median progression-free survival 18 months • Carboplatin with paclitaxel are commonly used • Can be repeated if relapse occurs after 6 months • Relapse within 6 months (platinum resistant disease), then 2nd line agents used: topotecan, liposomal, doxorubicin or etoposide (20% respond, progression-free survival 10 months).
Cervix cancer	• The role of chemo vs best supportive care has never been assessed in a clinical trial • Combination chemotherapy improves response rates and progression-free survival over single agent cisplatin, but offers no significant increase in overall survival • RRs for single agent cisplatin are ~20%, with PFS of 3–4 months and overall survival of 7–9 months • RRs for combination chemo are 25–35% with PFS of 4–5 months overall survival of 8–10 months • Combination regimens include agents such as cisplatin, ifosfamide, paclitaxel, bleomycin and topotecan

continued

CHEMOTHERAPY (Palliative)

Myeloma	• High dose chemotherapy with stem cell transplant for fit younger patients. Median survival 4–5 yrs. • Melphalan (or cyclophosphamide) and prednisolone offer 50% response (stable paraprotein levels for 24 months) • ABCM (doxorubicin, BCNU, cyclophosphamide, melphalan) has better response rate but greater toxicity and survival is not prolonged • Interferon alpha is sometimes used as maintenance therapy
Follicular Lymphoma	• Median survival is 8–10 years • Oral chlorambucil is used for symptomatic disease and 65% respond • Chemotherapy should be deferred until symptoms occur • Combination chemotherapy offers no survival benefit • 2nd line options include fludarabine (50%RR), CHOP, Rituximab (monoclonal antibody to CD20 receptor)
Head and neck cancer	• Cisplatin and 5–FU – 25–60% respond • Median survival 5–6 months
Soft tissue sarcomas	• Single agents (doxorubicin or ifosphamide) used – 30% respond • Response duration 6–12 months • Combination therapy offers no survival advantage, but improves response rates. Sometimes preferred for fit patients where bulk disease is causing symptoms • Chemo often produces significant toxicity
Malignant gliomas	• RRs with PCV or CCNU vary between 5–30% (better for Grade III astrocytomas than grade IV (glioblastoma)) • PCV better than CCNU alone for grade III astrocytomas. Probably equivalent for glioblastomas • Grade II and III oligodendrogliomas or oligoastrocytomas respond very well to PCV with 70% RR. • Temozolamide licensed as 2nd line, but poor response rates

Note: PCV = Procarbazine, CCNU and vincristine

Melanoma	<ul><li>Metastatic disease has a very poor prognosis – median survival 2–6 months</li><li>Single agents such as DTIC give 10–20% response, but for only 3–6 months</li><li>Higher response rates with chemo-immunotherapy (DTIC, interferon alpha and IL-2) at the expense of much higher toxicity</li></ul>

NOTES:

CR = *Complete response*, ie disappearance of all disease for at least 4 weeks (radiological, clinical, or pathological). *Partial response* means 50% decrease in tumour size and no progressive disease elsewhere for 4 weeks. *Stable disease* means increase of tumour of less than 25%. *Progressive disease* means more than 25% increase or new tumour sites.

The main goals of palliative chemotherapy are to improve symptom control, enhance quality of life and improve survival.

Toxicity of treatment is a major factor in decision making. Knowing when to stop chemotherapy is extremely important in order to avoid doing more harm than good.

Explain the aims of treatment very clearly *from the start*, and how and when decisions to continue or stop will be made.

Second and third line chemotherapy may be justified for some chemosensitive cancers e.g breast, ovary, small cell lung cancer.

SIDE EFFECTS OF CHEMOTHERAPY

- Nausea and vomiting
- Diarrhoea and constipation
- Myelosuppression
- Mucositis
- Fatigue and malaise, hepatitis
- Alopecia (reversible)
- Neurological (peripheral neuropathies, autonomic neuropathies, central neurological, ototoxicity)
- Cardiac (arrythmias, cardiac failure, coronary artery spasm)
- Urological (nephrotoxicity, haemorrhagic cystitis)
- Skin (erythema, pigmentation, extravasation)
- Pulmonary fibrosis (usually late effect)
- Infertility

COMPLEMENTARY THERAPIES

Aromatherapy	<ul><li>Frankincense, camomile, lavender and eucalyptus are all calming.</li><li>Usually combined with massage</li><li>Minute quantities of the oils are absorbed through the skin</li></ul>
Massage	<ul><li>Can reduce musculo-skeletal pains, headaches, migraine</li><li>Can reduce anxiety and pain (Corner 1994)</li><li>Reduces isolation. Provides a forum for ventilating feelings</li></ul>
Relaxation and visual imagery	<ul><li>Can decrease cancer pain (Syrjala et al 1995)</li><li>Deep relaxation can reduce anxiety and depression (Kite 1998)</li></ul>
Creative therapies (Art, Music, Writing, Reminiscence)	<ul><li>Can help patients understand their emotions</li><li>"I felt a strong inner compulsion to record what I was going through…and this has clarified my feeling and ideas" (a patient)</li></ul>
Acupuncture	<ul><li>Can reduce nausea and breathlessness, but less useful for pain</li><li>Traditional Chinese Medicine includes diet, meditation and herbal medicine</li></ul>
Hypnotherapy	<ul><li>Alters mood, sensation, and memory</li><li>Can reduce fears and increase self-control</li><li>Post-hypnotic suggestion can maintain "as if" feelings</li></ul>
Imagework	<ul><li>Uses images from the unconscious to enhance understanding of distress</li><li>e.g. "Imagine a picture of your experience at the moment – if the image could speak, what would it say?"</li><li>Powerful emotions may be released</li><li>Can restore peace of mind when other methods fail</li><li>Therapist requires training and support</li></ul>
Meditation	<ul><li>Increases calmness and inner peace</li><li>Can reduce worry and insomnia</li><li>Can be deepened by using bio-feedback</li><li>Elevates serotonin in the brain</li></ul>

COMPLEMENTARY THERAPIES

Homeopathy	• Detailed history of symptoms is taken • Can help stress and fatigue in some cancer patients • One substance is tried at a time (sucked not swallowed) • No side-effects (ultra-diluted substances) • 6c (six dilutions) or 30c (thirty dilutions) – 30c considered "stronger"
Herbal treatments (None proven effective)	• Iscador (mistletoe) • Jezentaihoto (Chinese hert) • Essiac (mixture of herbs) • Huang qi (root of milk vetch plant) • Hoxsey's herbs (cytotoxic in animals?) • Kombucha (derived from birch leaf tea)
Vitamins and minerals (None proven effective)	• High doses of vitamins A, C, E, retinoids and flavinoids • Hydrazine Sulphate • Selenium • Shark's cartilage • Shark-liver oil
Gerson Diet (Not effective)	• Developed by Max Gerson in the 1920s in Germany to treat TB • Organic juices (in large volumes), coffee enemas ("to eliminate toxins"), vaccine from patient's blood

NOTES:

Complementary therapies are person-centred approaches that can improve well being and help some patients to cope better. Orthodox medicine focuses on destroying cancer cells, complementary approaches focus on strengthening the internal environment. The immune system may be modulated by psychological interventions. (Walker, 1999)

Reassure your patient that adopting a complementary approach will not exclude them from conventional medical services.

Questions to consider: Does the Practitioner have recognized, current qualifications? Are they realistic about the outcome? Does it involve stopping conventional treatment? Are there any side-effects? Is it unpleasant or distressing to the patient? Is it very expensive? Are unrealistic claims for cure being made? Does it cause guilt (eg "they say I'm not trying hard enough")?

CONFUSION

Diagnosis Of Confusion (Usually obvious)	• Rapid onset (hours\days) • Disorientation (time\place\person) • Reduced awareness (of environment) • Easily startled • Rambling speech • Intellectual impairment • Poor short-term memory • Visual misperceptions • Paranoia • Fluctuates (worse in evenings) • Lucid intervals (better in mornings)
Consider Reversible Causes	• Drug-induced • Full bladder • Impacted faeces • Hypoxia • Brain metastases • Subdural haemorrhage • Heart Failure • UTI • Chest infection • Hypercalcaemia • Uraemia • Alcohol withdrawal (hallucinations) • Diazepam withdrawal • Hyponatraemia (SIADH)
Sedation	• May worsen confusion • Necessary if patient is frightened, agitated or may harm themselves or others. • eg haloperidol 10mg oral\IM • Midazolam 5–10mg IM can be added • Restraint, if the patient is violent, requires 3 professional carers
Quiet Environment	• Quiet, well-lit room • Avoid laughter in vicinity • Familiar staff – 1–2 trusted carers • Close relative may calm (may not)
Orientate Patient	• Wall clock – large • Avoid sudden changes • Explain all procedures • Introduce yourself each meeting • Remind patient of recent events ("I expect you remember.....")
Explanation	• Confusion is due to disease, not madness • Lucid intervals usually occur • Fears may relate to past, more than present

Support Family	• Confusion is a very distressing symptom for relatives • A relative may be needed to help manage the patient • Offer daily support
Monitor Mental State	• Useful to monitor improvement • Ask: "May I test your memory?" • eg "How many flowers\colours\cars can you remember?" • Record results

ANTI-PSYCHOTICS

		Dose		Sedation
levomepromazine	(Nozinan)	75–150mg	OD	++++
chlorpromazine	(Largactil)	25–50mg	TID	+++
haloperidol	(Serenace)	1–5mg	TID	+
olanzepine	(Zyprexa)	2.5–10mg	OD	+
respiridone	(Risperdal)	0.5–1mg	BD	+\–

NOTES:

Confusion (toxic delerium) is a common problem. Management is more effective if confusion is spotted early. Reversible factors may not be found by a "confusion screen" (examination, U&E, MSU, CXR) but correct management can still greatly reduce the the distress of patients and carers.

Drug doses that have been tolerated for months may suddenly become toxic as renal and hepatic function deteriorate.

Anti-psychotics (neuroleptics) cause emotional quietening and psychomotor slowing, without impairing the intellect. They are used short-term to quieten disturbed patients, with brain damage, toxic delerium, agitated depression or psychosis. At lower doses they are calming without causing too much sedation. Haloperidol has a high incidence of extra-pyridamidal side-effects.

The newer atypical anti-psychotics such as olanzepine and respiridone are very effective, and cause fewer movement disorders than the typical anti-psychotics, although parkinsonism can still occur.

NB Confusion is the most difficult symptom to cope with in the home – consider admission.

CONSTIPATION

ROUTINE LAXATIVES	
Lactulose 10–30ml BD or TID <u>with</u> **Senna** 1 nocte to 4 BD <u>or</u> Senna syrup 5–20ml BD	• Lactulose is too sweet for some, and can cause wind and distension. • Senna is stimulant
Co-danthramer (Codalax) 5–20ml BD	• 25 mg danthron\5 ml • Poloxamer as softener • stain wine red
Co-danthrusate (Normax) capsules 1–6 BD	• 50 mg danthron\capsule • Some patients prefer capsules
Co-danthramer forte 5–20ml BD	• 75mg danthron\5 ml
Liquid paraffin and magnesium hydroxide mixture (Milpar) 5–20ml BD <u>with</u> senna 1 nocte to 4 BD	• Useful for patients who dislike the above.
Polyethylene glycol (Movecol)	• Osmotic laxative • Oral powder, 1–2 sachets BD • 8 sachets in 1 litre of water can clear impacted faeces (use for up to 3 days) • Monitor electrolytes

STRONG LAXATIVES	
Picosulphate (Picolax)	• 1 sachet • Powerful stimulant • May cause abdominal cramps
Magnesium sulphate	• 10–20mls • Take with 1 pint water • Saline flusher • Diarrhoea after 3–6 hours

RECTAL MEASURES	
Glycerine suppositories	• Indicated if bowels not open for 3 days • Mainly a softener • Mildly stimulant
Bisacodyl Suppository (Dulcolax)	• Stimulant laxative • Acts in 1 hour • Can use with a glycerine suppository
Citrate Micro-enema (eg Microlette)	• 5mls • Slightly stronger than suppositories
Arachis oil Retention enema	• 130mls • Softens stools • Can be difficult to retain • Follow with phosphate enema
Phosphate enema	• 130mls • Stimulant – acts within 1 hour • Use soft catheter for colostomy
Digital disimpaction (rarely needed since movecol)	• Necessary for loaded rectum • Painful – sedate first • Follow with enemas • Abdominal massage helps to stimulate colon.

NOTES:

Daily laxatives are necessary for almost all patients on morphine (unless already liable to diarrhoea). Most need a softener and a stimulant. Increase doses as necessary every 1–2 days. 25% on laxatives still need rectal measures at times.

Stimulant laxatives act after 6–12 hours. Usually taken at night.

High-fibre diet is not tolerated by most ill patients. High fluid intake, fruit and fruit juice (especially prune juice) all help.

Bulking agents eg Fybogel 1–2 sachets a day, are not effective in preventing constipation but are useful in anal fissures. They should be taken with plenty of water.

Effects of chronic constipation: anorexia, malaise, colic, tenesmus, spurious diarrhoea, urinary retention, intestinal obstruction or mental confusion.

Abdominal masses that indent are faeces (not tumour). Abdominal Xray shows faeces in bowel (whereas in obstruction there are fluid levels).

COUGH

DRY COUGH	
Aspirate Pleural Effusion	• Effusion can present as dry cough • See Pleural Effusion
Radiotherapy	• Shrinks bronchial tumour (reduces cough in 40%).
Steroids	• eg dexamethasone 6–12mg daily • helpful for bronchial tumour or lung metastases • Reverses bronchospasm
Antitussives	• Codeine linctus 10ml 4 hourly – mild anti-tussive • Morphine is a strong anti-tussive • Methadone linctus (2mg in 5ml) 5–10ml nocte or TID, will sometimes control cough when morphine does not, but it accumulates (see Analgesics).
Bronchodilators	• Bronchospasm can present as drycough • Nebulized salbutamol 5mg 4 hourly • Nebulized ipratropium (Atrovent) 500 micrograms 4 hourly • Oral Phylocontin 225–450mg BD • Monitor with peak flow
Nebulized lignocaine	• 5ml 2%, used PRN • Especially effective for lung metastases • Pharyngeal numbness may occur • Avoid eating\drink for 20 minutes • Bronchospasm can occur (rarely)
Interpleural bupivacaine	• 20ml 0.5% bupivacaine 12 hourly • Epidural catheter in pleural space • Same side as lung disease. • Chest wall pain is also controlled

NOTES:

The cause of dry cough may be tumour mass, lung metastases, bronchospasm, pleural effusion or as a side-effect of ACE inhibitors.

Repeated coughing can cause insomnia, exhaustion, vomiting, rib fracture and cough syncope.

ACE inhibitors cause cough in 10–15% that can last 1–2 weeks after stopping. Angiotensin-II blockers (eg Losartan) have the same actions but do not cause the dry cough.

PRODUCTIVE COUGH	
Antibiotics	• Is sputum purulent? • Culture sputum • Add metronidazole for halitosis
Diuretics	• For heart failure (see notes)
Radiotherapy	• Controls haemoptysis in 90%
Nebulized saline	• Loosens tenacious sputum
Steam inhalations	• Loosen tenacious sputum
Mucolytics	• Loosens tenacious sputum • eg methylcysteine (Visclair) 100mg QID • Nebulized acetylycysteine (Parvolex) has been used
Physiotherapy	• Gentle percussion • Forced expirations ("huffing") • Loosens sputum and allows expectoration
Hyoscine hydrobromide	• Dries secretions • Useful for terminal phase, usually with diamorphine • 0.4mg IM, or • 1.2–3.6mg SC\24h
Suction	• Occasionally indicated in terminal phase if patient too weak to cough and distressed by tenacious sputum in throat • Use a soft catheter

NOTES:

Heart failure can cause cough, and can be of sudden onset following a myocardial infarction or arrythmia. Signs of left ventricular failure are tachycardia, triple rhythm, fine basal crepitations of pulmonary oedema, and pleural effusion. Signs of right ventricular failure are raised JVP, hepatomegaly and ankle and sacral oedema.

DENIAL

Is the family saying "Please don't tell"?
- Family denial is distressing (and tiring) because everyone fears saying the wrong thing
- Get the patient's permission to talk with the family
- Win the trust of the family by exploring their reasons for being so protective (see Family Meetings).
- Get their permission to talk to the patient
- Reassure them you will not give the patient any unrequested information, but explain that as a professional you cannot lie
- Give the patient the opportunity to ask questions
- Talk with the patient and family together.

What does the patient understand?
- If you ask "What do you understand about your illness" many patients respond by saying "I don't understand anything". This is a self-protective response.
- If you continue to explore their understanding by holding a conversation about their illness, eg "And what happened next?" and "So what did the doctors explain at that point?" it begins to become clearer how much they understand and whether they are really in denial.

Do they have any questions?
- "Denial" may simply be misinterpretation due to a lack of opportunities to ask questions about their illness.

Is the denial doing any harm?
- Denial is a normal and protective defence, simply one form of the selective attention that we all use every day to concentrate, think and function
- If denial is not causing anxiety or communication difficulties, denial can be left unchallenged, as a defence that is working
- Some patients adjust and deal with all the relevant practical matters then prefer to pretend it is not happening ("non-attention denial" or wise acceptance)

Negotiate how much information is wanted
- Ask: "Would it be helpful to have more information about your illness?"
- Acknowledge that asking questions can feel frightening (because of what you might say and what they might hear).
- Explain that more understanding can reduce uncertainty and fear

Responding to fixed denial
- Never give unrequested information (which causes anxiety or anger or both)
- Use optimism. The expression "I hope…" can convey support without being confrontational, dishonest or colluding ("I hope that you have been cured too…")

> **Monitor the denial**
> - Ask at each visit : "How do you feel things are going at the moment?"
> - As the patient feels more secure and trusting they may be able to ask for more information.
> - Ask: "Do you ever feel frightened?"
> - Addressing and discussing the truth reduces fear, but the fear tends to be replaced by appropriate sadness and grief.

NOTES:

Denial is a psychological defence that can be useful as well as harmful, and needs to be respected as an important way of coping with fear. Denial should not be used as a perjorative term to describe patients who are somehow "unable to face the truth".

Excessive denial however, often causes a lot of distress by preventing the person making important adjustments and appropriate plans for the future. It can also cause a lot of family distress, because important conversations cannot happen. This is the sort of denial that needs gently challenging by building trust and then asking questions.

Denial feels uncomfortable for professionals because they are being asked to collude with an unreal fantasy. Denial is an unconscious defence – and therefore not amenable to logical discussion. "Bargaining" is a form of partial denial eg "I will only accept this illness if —— happens".

Denial can be intermittent. Some patients who have accepted their situation may still appear to "deny" it at other times (eg inappropriately planning holidays abroad) in order to have a rest from all the exhausting emotions. This partial or intermittent denial is normal, and it is the <u>inability</u> of some patients to use denial in this way that causes them to be severely anxious, because they cannot stop thinking about their illness.

Non-attention to the disease can mimic denial. Do not mistake wise acceptance for denial. *"I have a life-threatening illness. What I find interesting is how I can spend most of my time not thinking about my prognosis. This does not make me avoid reasonable planning for the future".* (Arthur Rifkin, psychiatrist "Is it denial or wisdom to accept life threatening illness" BMJ 3 Nov 2001.)

DEPRESSION

Criteria for Depressive illness (DSM-IV)

5 symptoms daily for at least 2 weeks

Main symptoms (at least one)
- Depressed mood
- Loss of interest\pleasure

Additional symptoms
- Altered sleep (early waking)
- Change in appetite
- Loss of energy
- Ideas of self-harm
- Feeling worthless\guilty
- Poor concentration
- Agitation (or retardation)

Appropriate sadness or depressive illness?

The following suggest depressive illness:

- Low mood persists longer than 2 weeks
- Inability to smile or greet relatives
- Low self-esteem
- Pathological crying
- Recurrent thoughts of death

SSRIs
Eg citalopram 20mg OD

- First-line anti-depressant
- Take 2–4 weeks for effect
- May cause nausea
- 80% are helped
- Mirtazapine 15–30mg ON is useful for palliative care(dual action on both serotonin and noradrenegric receptors, increases appetite, sedating and no drug interactions)

Tricyclics
Eg Amitriptyline 50–150mg ON

- May be preferred if there is also:
    - Nausea
    - Insomnia
    - Drooling
    - Neuropathic pain
- Anti-cholinergic side-effects (dry mouth, blurred vision, retention)
- Dothiepin and lofepramine cause fewer side-effects

St John's Wort
- Herbal remedy
- Available OTC (over the counter)
- Effective for mild depression

Psychostimulants
eg methylphenidate 5–30mg BD
eg dexamfetamine 5–10mg BD

- Effective for mild depression due to physical illness
- Widely used in US
- Rapid onset, 1–2 days
- Well tolerated
- Not addictive, but tolerance occurs

Cognitive therapy
- Developed 1979 by Aaron Beck
- Negative view of self, negative interpretations of events, pessimism and distorted thinking (eg "disasterization") cause depresssion
- Therapist teaches person to identify and challenge their negative thoughts and assumptions.
- 12–20 sessions + homework
- Proven effectiveness for depression

Refer to Psychiatrist

Consider if severe with phobia, delusions or marked withdrawal (eg refusal to talk)

ECT
- Electro-convulsive therapy (described 1938)
- Effective for severe depression resistant to anti-depressants
- Equipment is portable
- GA+Muscle relaxants – safe in frail or with bone metastases
- Improvement can be rapid (1–2 weeks)

NOTES:

Depressive illness occurs in 10% of patients in Palliative Care, and is more likely to respond to anti-depressants plus emotional support than to either one alone. Appropriate sadness due to losses causes low mood ("depression") for 1–2 weeks but does not cause low self-esteem and responds to counselling and social support.

The physical features of depressive illness (anorexia, loss of energy) are also common in cancer, so are less helpful in diagnosis.

Anti-depressants are underused in Palliative Care, or given "too little too late" for many patients. SSRIs are now first line treatment, with few side effects. Citalopram causes less nausea than the other SSRIs. Venlafaxine and mertazepine are both useful SSRIs. Mirtazepine is one of the few anti-depressants that increases appetite. Tricyclics still have a role as anti-depressants, especially when night sedation is also needed.

DIABETES

Diagnosis	• Random blood glucose above 11 mmol\l.
Causes	• Known diabetic • Steroid-induced • CA pancreas • Ectopic ACTH (small cell CA bronchus)
Symptoms of diabetes:	• Thirst • Polyuria • Drowsiness • Weakness • Recurrent thrush.
Aim of treatment	• Blood glucose 7–12 mmol/l • To avoid hypoglycaemia or symptomatic hyperglycaemia
Gliclazide (Diamicron)	• Short acting oral hypoglycaemic • Boosts insulin secretion • 80mg tablet, scored • 40–80–160mg with breakfast • Up to 160mg BD
Starting insulin	• Actrapid TID (units by sliding scale) • Mixtard 30 is useful to reduce number of injections • Warn about hypoglycaemia (sweating, tremor, altered behaviour) • Patient should carry sugar
Diet	• Can be relaxed • Sugar allowable in moderation • Spread carbohydrate over the day • Some diabetics prefer to maintain strict diet
Starting steroids in diabetics	• Steroids increase blood glucose, but potential benefits often outweigh diabetic risks • Insulin requirements increase • Patients on hypoglycaemic drugs may need to change to insulin • Monitor carefully – consider admission
Vomiting	• Change to soluble insulin (eg Actrapid) TID • Give according to a "sliding scale":

DIABETES

Sliding scale	Blood Glucose (mmol\l)		Soluble Insulin eg Actrapid	
(Measure	<10	give	0	units
glucose TID	10–15	give	6	units
before meals)	15–22	give	10	units
	>22	give	20	units
Terminal phase	• Mixtard 30, 6 units BD is safe even if eating little or nothing • Monitoring is not necessary • Insulin can be stopped if the patient is unconscious.			

NOTES:

Steroids may induce diabetes, and this is quite a common situation in Palliative Care, because steroids are often used to control symptoms. Steroids are commonly given as a single dose in the morning (to avoid insomnia) and the blood sugar then often rises highest in the evenings. If this pattern occurs a single dose of Mixtard 30 can be given before lunch, possibly adding some Actrapid in the evening.

Strict diabetic control (which is intended to prevent long-term microvascular complications) is no longer necessary. Aiming to keep glucose below 15mmol\1 is sufficient.

Dosages of oral hypoglycaemic and insulin often need to be reduced gradually as weight loss occurs, to avoid hypoglycaemia.

Mixtard-30 contains 30% soluble insulin and 70% isophane insulin. Isophane insulin is longer acting, with peak effect at 4–7 hours, and lasting 12–16 hours.

Insulin glargine (Lantus) is a new once a day insulin injection that releases insulin slowly over 24 hours and gives a very useful background treatment, with little risk of hypoglycaemia when used alone. It can be given with gliclazide or soluble insulin if necessary. Start with 8 units daily and increase every 4 days by 2–4 units.

Metformin is best avoided because it commonly causes nausea when first started and because it can cause lactic acidosis.

The newer oral hypoglycaemics such as acarbose (which reduces absorbtion of sugar) and the glitazones (which reduce insulin resistance) are rarely necessary in the palliative care setting.

Patients who have been diabetic for years will have tried to maintain very careful control, and may feel it is "giving up too soon" if told they can relax their control. Discuss their attitudes towards their diabetes. Some patients (and their relatives) may feel better psychologically to know that strict control of glucose levels willl continue as normal. Others may be pleased to know they can be more relaxed about it. Avoid assumptions – ask!

DIARRHOEA

Drug-induced diarrhoea?	• Antibiotics • NSAIDs • Cytotoxics • Iron
Disimpact rectum	• Impacted faeces cause spurious diarrhoea (see notes) • Disimpact (see Constipation)
Adjust laxatives	• Intermittant (excessive) laxative use is a common problem • Stress daily use and titrate dose
Loperamide	• 2–4mg QID • Most effective anti-diarrhoeal • For diarrhoea due to abdominal malignancy or malignant intestinal dysfunction (see Intestinal obstruction)
Creon	• For Steatorrhoea (see notes) • Pancreatic enzyme supplement • 2–4 capsules with meals (1 with snacks) • Effect increased by reducing gastric acid secretion
Rectal steroids	• eg Colifoam enema BD (125mg hydrocortisone per application) • Radiation proctitis • Discharge from rectal tumour
Octreotide	• SC 200–600mcg\24hr • Reduces GI secretions and motility (see Intestinal Obstruction) • Reduces 5HT secretion of Carcinoid tumours (diarrhoea, flushing, wheezing) • Reduces diarrhoea due to malignant entero-colic fistula
Desmopressin	• Reduces renal production of urine • Useful if urine is passing PR (recto-vesical fistula) • 100–300mcg PO nocte to start
Gastrostomy feed	• Concentrated feed can cause diarrhoea • Dilute by 50%
Oral electrolytes	• eg Dioralyte • Indicated for dehydration
Antibiotics	• Infective? – send stool cultures • Discuss treatment with lab

Transanal surgery	• Resection\Cryo\Laser • For CA rectum in situ • Reduces discharge
Defunctioning colostomy	• For recto-vaginal fistula
Bowel regulation	• Constipate then clear bowel with enema 2–3 times\week • Used to control loose motions as a last resort, eg faecal incontinence due to loss of sphincter control.
Bulking agents	• eg Fybogel BD • Useful for colostomy regulation • Helps to produce a formed motion in rectal tumours with discharge

NOTES:

Spurious diarrhoea is a late complication of impacted faeces, and means small amounts of watery stools, often with some faecal incontinence, following a long period of constipation, and it is usually suspected from the history.

Steatorrhoea means loose, fatty stools which are foul-smelling and float. Diarrhoea occurs 4–5 times a day, unaffected by standard anti-diarrhoeal drugs. The common cause is malabsorbtion of fat due to blockage of the pancreatic duct by tumour. It responds quickly to pancreatic replacement, eg Creon.

Loperamide is the most effective anti-diarrhoeal. It tends to be under-used in diarrhoea due to abdominal malignancy for fear of causing constipation. It there is troublesome diarrhoea – treat it.

Other causes of diarrhoea include diet (eg spices), malignant bowel disease (see Intestinal Obstruction) ulcerative colitis, ileal resection (when bile salts are not absorbed, causing malabsorbtion), Carcinoid tumours, panceatic islet cell tumours secreting gastrin (treated with ranitidine) and diabetic neuropathy.

Diarrhoea in AIDS may be due to cryptosporidium, CMV (treated with gancyclovir), salmonella, MAI or KS. In culture-negative diarrhoea a trial of ciprofloxacin or metronidazole may be indicated. Octreotide can be effective if anti-diarrhoeals are not.

DRUG INTERACTIONS

Baclofen	• Tricyclics potentiate effect
Carbamazepine	• Reduces effect of steroids by 50% • Toxicity may occur with co-proxamol, erythromycin, verapamil, fluoxetine, diltiazem.
Cholestyramine and Colestipol	• Reduce absorption of most drugs • Take 1 hour after (or 4 hours before) all drugs
Dantrolene	• Verapamil may cause hyperkalaemia
Dexamethasone	• Possible increased GI effects of NSAIDs • Carbamazepine and phenytoin reduce effect by 50% • Possible hypokalaemia with frusemide
Dextropro-poxyphene	• Enhances carbamazepine • Enhances warfarin
Fluconazole	• Phenytoin levels rise • Warfarin levels rise
Fluoxetine	• Increases extrapyramidal effects of haloperidol
Haloperidol	• Carbamazepine reduces effect • Metoclopramide may worsen side-effects (dystonia)
Ketoconazole	• Antacids, H2 blockers, omeprazole all reduce absorption
Levomepromazine	• MAOIs – sudden death reported
Metronidazole	• Phenytoin levels rise • Alcohol can cause headache\flushing
Midazolam	• Erythromycin can potentiate
Morphine	• MAOIs – hypertensive crisis
NSAIDs	• Warfarin and digoxin potentiated • Lithium levels rise • Methotrexate toxicity • Steroids may increased GI effect
Omeprazole	• Reduces absorption of ketoconazole
Octreotide	• Insulin may be potentiated

DRUG INTERACTIONS

Ranitidine	• Reduces absorption of ketoconazole
Spironolactone	• Avoid potassium salts • Avoid with other potassium-sparing diuretics: amiloride, triamterene • NSAIDs and ACE-inhibitors increase risk of hyperkalaemia • Digoxin is potentiated
Sucralfate	• Reduces absorption of warfarin, and phenytoin
Terfenadine	• Erythromycin, frusemide, tricyclics and anti-psychotics can cause arrhythmias
Tricyclics	• MAOIs – excitation, hypertension • Terfenadine and astemizole – arrhythmias
Warfarin	• Potentiated by dextropropoxyphene, NSAIDs, quinidine, omeprazole, tamoxifen, flutamide, ketoconazole, fluconazole, metronidazole, co-trimoxazole, chloramphenicol, ciprofloxacin, stanozolol and fosphamide.

NOTES:

Drug interactions are ESPECIALLY common with *warfarin* and the *anticonvulsants* – check very carefully when prescribing these drugs. Another drug which causes important interactions is *amiodarone* (for atrial fibrillation) which can cause fatal arrhythmias with tricyclics, phenothiazines, haloperidol, quinine or erythromycin.

Always check for drug interactions when prescribing.

The commonest cause of drug interactions is competition for liver enzymes.

DYSPHAGIA

Assessment	• Difficulty with solids? • Difficulty with liquids? • Pain on swallowing? • Pain with hot drinks (thrush)? • lip closure (say 'PA') • tongue movement (say 'KA') • NB Observe swallowing • Oral-pharyngeal transit time? • Choking? (neurological) • Coughing? (fistula)

MANAGEMENT OF MALIGNANT STRICTURES

Radiotherapy	• For squamous cancers of oesophagus • External or intraluminal • Dysphagia recurs in 60% • RT can precede or follow tube insertion
Oesophageal tube	• For unresectable tumours • Improves swallowing in 90% • Fizzy drink after meals.
Self-expanding metal stents	• Advance over tubes • Fit through smaller strictures • Expand wider than tubes • Lower re-obstruction rate • Made of 'memory metal' • Mesh incorporates into oesophagus wall
Oesophageal dilation	• Can improve swallowing for a time if intubation or stenting fails • Following oesophagectomy 30% need repeated dilation of the anastomosis
Laser	• Improves swallowing in 90%. • Can be repeated every 4–6 weeks • Not for extrinsic compression of the oesophagus by mediastinal nodes.
Steroids	• Dexamethasone 8–12mg\24h SC • Effective for dysphagia in oesophageal or head and neck tumours. • Reduces peri-tumour oedema • 50% get relief in 1–2wks
NG tube	• Indicated for short-term management of neurological dysphagia or cough due to a tracheo-oesophage fistula. • See Gastrostomy.
Gastrostomy (PEG)	• Indicated for hunger/thirst • See Gastrostomy

GENERAL MEASURES	
Anti-fungals	• Fluconazole 50mg OD • Oesophageal thrush causes dysphagia • It typically causes pain with hot drinks • It can be severe even with no oral thrush
Maalox with 2% Lignocaine 50:50 mixture	• 10ml hourly • Relieves pain of radiation oesophagitis • (Mucaine no longer available)
Strong Short-acting Analgesia	• Visceral ache when eating • Give extra analgesia 20 min before meals • Eg dextromoramide 5mg sublingually • Eg Actiq lozenge (see Fentanyl)
Scopaderm Patch	• Transdermal hyoscine hydrobromide • 0.5 mg/72 hours • Reduces dribbling in severe dysphagia • 2 patches may be needed
Antibiotics	• Aspiration can cause RTI • Aspiration may be silent • Is RTI a terminal event? • Discuss with patient (?)
Diamorphine Hyoscine	• Terminal phase, to control secretions and cough (see Terminal Phase)
Neurological dysphagia	• eg Motor Neurone Disease • Suck ice • Ice-pack on throat • Speech\swallowing therapist • Palatal plate • Crico-pharnygeal myotomy • NG tube\PEG

NOTES:

The commonest causes of dysphagia are malignant stricture and oesophageal thrush (which typically causes burning discomfort after hot drinks). Benign peptic stricture can still occur!

Neurological dysphagia is most commonly a problem in MND Neck position and food consistency become very important. Involve a dietician and a swallowing therapist to give advice. If the patient becomes thirsty or hungry or is troubled by nasal regurgitation, choking or aspirating, then a gastrostomy may be indicated – discuss carefully with the patient. The oro-pharyngeal transit time can be assessed by putting a hand over the patients neck as they swallow, and it is the time between the floor of the mouth tightening and the larynx moving up and down – normally about a second. If it is prolonged to 4–5 seconds a gastrostomy may be indicated.

EMERGENCIES

PSYCHOLOGICAL:	
Panic attacks	<ul><li>Terrifying for the patient.</li><li>Lorazepam 1mg sublingually PRN</li><li>Propranolol 20–40mg QID</li><li>Counselling and support</li><li>Consider admission</li></ul>
Agitation	<ul><li>Fear\Pain\Hypoxia\Full bladder</li><li>Sedation if the patient is in danger of hurting themself or others</li><li>IM 10mg Haloperidol</li></ul>

RADIOTHERAPY:	
Spinal cord compression	<ul><li>Dexamethasone 16mg immediately Radiotherapy – same day</li></ul>
SVC compression	<ul><li>Usually of gradual onset</li><li>Steroids, RT or chemotherapy</li><li>Oxygen for acute dyspnoea (poor prognosis)</li><li>IV frusemide</li><li>SVC stent</li><li>Anti-coagulation if CT scan shows thrombosis (sudden onset)</li></ul>

SURGICAL:	
Acute urinary retention	<ul><li>Catheterize</li><li>Suprapubic catheter for urethral obstruction</li><li>Consider repeat TURP</li></ul>
Fractures	<ul><li>Xray to confirm</li><li>Is it pathological or traumatic?</li><li>Analgesia (if painful)</li><li>Immobilize by splint or skin traction</li><li>Internal fixation if possible</li></ul>
Stridor	<ul><li>Tracheal compression</li><li>Oxygen or helium\oxygen</li><li>IV dexamethasone 16mg</li><li>IV Frusemide (if SVC compression)</li><li>RT\laser</li><li>Emergency stent (via endoscope)</li><li>Emergency tracheostomy</li><li>Sedation if a terminal event</li></ul>

MEDICAL:		
Severe pain	•	Constant attention until pain controlled
	•	? Fracture
	•	? Urinary retention
	•	? Colic – Buscopan needed
	•	SC 2.5mg diamorphine
Haemorrhage	•	Constant attention
	•	May be a terminal event
	•	Midazolam 5–15mg IM into the deltoid if distressed (S/C not absorbed?)
	•	IVI, X-match only if appropriate
Acute breathlessness	•	100% oxygen
	•	SC midazolam 1–5mg
	•	IV or SC diamorphine
Fits	•	Diazepam PR (Stesolid) 10–40mg
Hypercalcaemia	•	IV fluids and IV biphosphonates
	•	Sedation may be appropriate if it is a terminal event

DRUGS:		
Allergic reaction	•	IV hydrocortisone 100mg
	•	IV piriton 10mg
Dystonic reaction	•	Occurs with metoclopramide haloperidol or phenothiazines
	•	Causes tongue stiffness/abnormal movements
	•	Reverses dramatically with IV benztropine 1mg
	•	May take several days to wear off completely
Morphine overdose (very rare)	•	IV naloxone 100–200 mcg

NOTES:

Calm explanation of events to patient and family is an essential part of managing an emergency.

Many emergencies can be avoided by anticipation and planning ahead. If an event is expected and prepared for (practically <u>and</u> psychologically) it is less of an "emergency".

See <u>Appendix</u> for useful drugs for palliative care emergencies.

EMOTIONAL DISTRESS

CLOSED RESPONSES	EMOTION	OPEN RESPONSE	HOW TO FACILITATE COPING
• Detachment • Fantasy thinking • "Bargaining" • Manic activity • Avoiding conversations • Inability to make appropriate plans.	⇐ Denial ⇒	Facing reality	Build trust until they feel safe enough to ask questions (see Denial) Encourage communication (see Family meetings)
• Blaming others • Being withdrawn • Acting on impulse • Aggressive humour • Projection	⇐ Anger ⇒	Fighting the illness	Allowing ventilation of anger, explore underlying feelings, re-direct the energy
• Feeling miserable • Crying • Living in the past • Ruminating on losses	⇐ Sadness ⇒	Grieving and adjustment	Empathic conversations – that identify and explore the meaning of the losses being experienced.
• Helplessness • Feeling out of control • Not taking responsibility • Avoiding decisions • Being childlike	⇐ Dependency ⇒	Participating in care	Give support during the "helpless" phase then re-engage the patient in their own care
• Obsessional worrying • Anxious pre-occupation with illness or drugs • Hypochondria • Paranoia	⇐ Fear ⇒	Realistic daily coping	Build trust, teach relaxation and visualization offer diversional activities and use cognitive approaches (see Depression)

CLOSED RESPONSES	EMOTION	OPEN RESPONSE	HOW TO FACILITATE COPING
• "Why me?" • "What's the point?" • Fear of "not existing" • Guilt about the past	⇐ Hopelessness ⇒	Searching for meaning	Discuss spiritual aspects of being ill, sublimate distress into positive actions, helping others in some way, move towards acceptance (see Spiritual Distress)

NOTES:

This is a practical, task-orientated model of the emotional responses to dying that points to ways of helping – by encouraging open responses. It builds on Kubler-Ross's 1969 description of denial, anger, bargaining, depression and acceptance which was a very helpful insight and enabled doctors to understand how to draw alongside dying patients. Kubler-Ross demonstrated that patients actually felt *better* when enabled to talk honestly about their feelings – a revolutionary idea at the time.

Emotional distress is normal during serious illness (or any major life change). Coping involves dealing with emotions, while simultaneously trying to seek information and make decisions.

People vary in their resources (inner and outer) but encouraging a shift towards more open responses can facilitate coping. Openness in one area tends to facilitate openness in other areas. Willingness to shift to a more open coping response is more likely around the time of a crisis ("I just can't cope at the moment – something will have to change").

Good copers tend to have more open responses, to be optimistic, resourceful, willing to express feelings, knowledgeable about their illness, socially well supported and to have a sense of purpose and realistic short-term goals.

Closed responses are not necessarily harmful. Each of the closed responses (psychological defenses) can be effective at times, enabling the person to cope at a certain points in their illness, but they are more likely to become maladaptive and to increase distress, or to result in anxiety or depression, in which case they may need to be challenged.

EQUIPMENT

Mobility	• Walking frame\rollator • Raised toilet seat • Handrails\ ramps • Non-slip bath mats • Chair cushion elevator • Stairlift • High trolley (to move things) • Wheelchair
Eating	• 2–handled beaker • Combined spoon-knife • Non-slip table mats • Flexible straws • Flask (for hot\cold drinks)
Kitchen equipment	• High stool • Liquidizer • Microwave • Ice maker • Electric tin opener • Jar opener
Continence	• Bedpans • Urine bottles • Incontinence sheaths • Penis pouches • Catheter bags • Plastic mattress cover • Commode
Nursing	• Drug card (see Prescribing) • Medicine spoons\syringes • Mouth swabs (foamsticks) • Handling slings • Hoist • Colostomy bags (leaking wounds) • Nappi-sack deodourized bags for soiled dressings
Skin care	• Moisturizing cream • Chair cushion • Heel\elbow pads • Foam mattress cover • Air-wave mattress • Bath seat (jelly cushion)
Bed comfort	• Light bedding (e.g. Duvet) • Trapeze/"monkey pole" • Jacob's ladder (pull on, to sit) • Leg cradle

Bed comfort (continued)	● V-pillow ● Tissues and basin ● Back rest eg Matchett bag ● Armrest for oedematous arm ● eg Matchett bag ● Recliner chair instead of bed?
Bedroom Facilities	● Bedside table ● Bedside light ● Electric fan ● Call bell\hand bell ● TV (remote-control) ● Portable phone

NOTES:

Timing is important when it comes to offering and providing equipment. If it is offered too early it can be frightening and demoralizing ("I don't want to get to the stage of needing to use that sort of thing"). If it is offered too late it can increase suffering and frustration ("Why didn't anyone think of giving us this help before?"). One skill of the professional team is to offer equipment in a timely way.

ETHICAL PROBLEMS

Is the patient competent to make a decision?	• Can they retain information? • If not, decision is based on what patient would want. • Next of kin may need to witness decision
Does the patient need a spokesperson?	• Can the patient communicate? • Did the patient write a 'Living Will' (advanced directive)
Will the treatment benefit the patient?	• Treatment that has no hope of giving physical or psychological benefit is unethical (side-effects and waste of limited resources).
Will it do harm?	• Most treatments have potential side-effects • Explain risks
Will benefit outweigh harm?	• This may be unknown • Discuss a trial of treatment • If benefit does not occur (or ceases) will treatment be stopped?
What if the patient refuses the treatment?	• A patient is allowed to refuse any treatment (even if this endangers their life) • The patient's wishes take precedence over the family's wishes
What if the patient requests a harmful treatment?	• The doctor also has autonomy and can refuse to give a treatment that he/she believes would do more harm than good.
Am I being prejudiced?	• Is my treatment ever different? • What if the patient were younger? My age? My colour? My nationality? My class? My profession?
Have I gathered all the relevant data?	• What do the rest of the medical team think? • Have I attempted to see an alternative point of view? • What do the relatives think? • Data-gathering reduces the risk of individual prejudice affecting the decision.
What will the consequences be?	• The consequences may be uncertain • This needs honest discussion with the patient (or family if the patient is incompetent)

Who will really benefit?	• What are the real motives behind giving this treatment? • Is it really to please the relatives\nurses\doctors?
Who holds the power to make the decision?	• The person with the power (and responsibility) may be making the wrong decision. • Can they be challenged?

NOTES:

Ethical problems usually arise when an unusual situation makes the right course of action difficult to see. Generally we do not need to think too deeply about most of our day-to-day clinical decisions, because they are based on well-tried assumptions which work. It is only when we meet a situation that is new, and in which the consequences of a wrong decision may be serious, that we have to carefully consider the options with the patient, and the pros and cons of each option, and choose the best course of action. Patients find it easier to make decisions if they know they can change their minds.

The 4 main principles of Medical Ethics are:
1 Respect autonomy
2 Do good
3 Do no harm
4 Decisions should be socially just (eg the use of scarce resources for a minimal benefit may not be justified).

The main difficulty is this: no set of principles can guarantee a correct decision. Often there is no right or wrong answer to a problem. Often we cannot be certain that benefit will outweigh harm. The important thing is *the way* the decision is reached. Is the patient competent to make the decision? Can the patient communicate? Has the patient been given accurate information in an unbiased way and a way they can understand? Does the patient understand the explanation of the various options? Have they been given time to discuss them? Has everyone been consulted who should have been? Have uncertainty and risk been explained clearly? Have these efforts to reach the correct decision been documented in the notes?

CASE STUDY

A married woman of 50 has far-advanced cancer of the cervix that has caused a lot of pain in the recent past. She has suddenly become very confused. She has been feeling quite well for the past month, and is still the main carer for her handicapped daughter aged 13. She wrote a living will 3 years ago. It states she would not want her life prolonging in the event of a terminal complication. She is found to have bilateral ureteric obstruction. Her husband, who is a vet, is adamant that ureteric stents should be inserted. What would you do?

FAMILY MEETINGS 1

Ask the patient's permission

- Ask: "Would you like me to meet with your family?"
- Ask: "Do you want to be present at the meeting?"
- NB Do not talk to the family without the patient's permission
- Who is "family" for this patient

Plan the meeting (This is a skill in itself)

- Who invites who?
- When should it happen? (avoid rushing)
- Where will it happen?
- Who will want to be there from the family?
- Which professionals will attend?
- Does it need to happen in stages? (meet some, then others, then all together?)

Prepare the room

- Book the room (so the meeting is free of interruptions)
- Quiet room with enough chairs
- Warm and ventilated
- No phones
- Toys, paper and coloured pens
- Have tissues ready

Greet the family

- Say hello to everyone in the room
- "Break the ice" eg "how was your journey"?
- Say who you are and explain your role
- Ask: "Is anyone missing from the family today?"

Set clear time boundaries

- Eg "we have an hour together now"
- Eg "We can decide at the end if we need to meet again"
- Eg "We have five minutes left"

Start the discussion

- Explain the value of family meetings (eg "family ties people together, and I am sure this illness is affecting you all in different ways").
- Talk with the patient first (if present)
- Update the situation for the benefit of family members
- Ask each person: "What is the most difficult thing for you at the moment? THIS IS THE KEY STAGE
- Don't leave anyone out

Explain the needs of children

- Children of ALL ages need information and explanation
- Children are NOT protected by being left out
- The parents must decide how and when to tell them ("you know your children far better than us, but what experts know very clearly is that children of all ages cope much better later on, if they are included by the family, given plenty of age-appropriate explanations and given opportunities to ask questions and to be curious")
- Suggest letting teachers know about the situation

Offer availability

- Further explanation may be needed later
- Consider offering to meet others in the family, eg grandparents

Document the meeting in the clinical notes

- Those who attended
- Draw (or add to) the family tree
- List key issues
- Summarise significant conversations
- Note any decisions

NOTES:

Family meetings should be a routine part of assessment in all hospices and palliative care settings, and especially if there are children in the family. They SAVE A LOT OF TIME, not only in terms of information-giving to a group (rather than repeatedly to individual relatives) but also because they build trust, allow feelings to be ventilated, reduce anxiety and enable families to support themselves better.

A single meeting, especially at a time of crisis, is often enough to strengthen relationships solve problems and find new energy for the future. Patients usually welcome the idea – they are often concerned about their relatives.

A specific invitation is important ("We would like to meet with you and your family – would that be helpful"). Even if it is initially refused, the invitation itself is a significant message about family-centred care, and it can be offered again. The visit of family members from far away provides a useful opportunity for a renewed invitation.

End with affirmation and honest praise. ("You have had the courage to face up to the worst and this can make you stronger together" or "You have coped so well up to now"). This greatly increases the effectiveness of the meeting.

FAMILY MEETINGS 2

FURTHER NOTES

1. **Learn how to convene and conduct a family meeting** – it is a VERY useful skill. It can feel threatening to meet a whole family, but with a bit of practice it is straightforward and always very helpful. Work in partnership with a colleague to start with.

2. **Setting a date for a family meeting** a few days ahead can be a useful strategy for families with communication difficulties, to prompt some discussion before the meeting takes place ("What will we talk about?").

3. **Family meetings are a strange experience** for many modern families, who may rarely sit down and talk together (free of TV and computer interruptions). Simply holding a family meeting is surprisingly effective. As painful subjects are shared, tension is released.

4. **Think of the family as a resource group** and as experts in their own problems ("have any of you experience of this sort of situation before?").

5. **Be a catalyst**. Your role is mainly to encourage the family to meet together. "Families that are brought together, will talk together". Don't feel you have to interrupt when they start having a lively discussion – let them.

6. **The aim** is to gently work towards increasing openness within the family. Professionals sometimes unwittingly worsen family communication by the incompetent breaking of bad news ("The doctor told us not to tell him").

7. **Be open and factual**. Give information in a straightforward way. Use factual terminology. Avoid euphemisms such as "passing away", which reduce openness and imply that it is dangerous to speak directly about death (and therefore the family should not either). Being open provides a model for the family to copy.

8. **Find out what the family know** before giving any explanations. There is often a spokesperson but it is always worth asking "Is that what everyone else was thinking"?

9. **It boosts a family's confidence** to know they are in partnership with the professionals ("you all know her best – it would be very helpful to have your thoughts about the problem").

10. **Respect the hope for life**. Remain as optimistic as possible. Be sure you know something about the patient and their life before they were ill. It is insensitive to discuss death before discussing life.

11. **Establish at least one open relationship**. If the family are colluding in denial, identify the person who seems most comfortable with being open, and gently explore that person's experience, so the rest of the family can witness a different sort of open discussion ("Have you known anyone else with cancer?"). This can have a powerful effect in normalizing the family's way of coping.

12. **Remain calm**. The family is already stressed and will not be helped by further upset. Your own emotions (sadness, anger) need to be controlled. Remind yourself that their situation is not your situation. Discuss your own feelings later, with a colleague.

13. **Families vary** enormously (single parent, divorced, step-families, re-constituted ("blended") families, extended, fostered, communal, gay). Do not assume all families are like your own family. Draw a family tree.

14. **A family is emotionally interdependent**. A family is like a decorative mobile – touch one bit and the whole system moves. It helps to remind a family of this (eg "This problem must be affecting you all").

15. **A family has a past**. Family responses are more easily understood when previous losses are explored.

16. **A family has a life cycle**, characterized by change (new school, new job, adolescence, marriage, new in-laws, a new baby, house moves, "empty nest", retirement). A terminal illness may co-incide with other problems or crises in the family – find out *what else* is happening for them.

17. **A family has shared ideas**. Use the family's words and phrases, at least to start with, before introducing new words. ("I knew he had a tumour but now you're telling me its cancer."). Avoid premature interpretations of a family's behaviour, which can rightly cause anger. Affirm their strengths ("You have cared for him so well.") and they will volunteer their weaknesses.

18. **A family has a future together**, it is a living system with a dying member, but the system will go on. Helping the patient and family discuss the future together helps them do their grieving together. It reduces their isolation and gives the dying person a part in the family's future eg a spouse discussing the future care of the children, or teaching household roles and skills. Bereaved people always find it a comfort to have discussed the future with the person who died.

19. **The way a family supports children** around the time of a death will affect their future attitudes to losses and crises. *"We are not just dealing with present problems...we are modelling ways of coping with future living"*. Working with families around the time of a death to help them communicate to their children is effective preventive psychiatry.

20. **Avoid asking "How do you feel"**. Ask about events (eg "What might happen if —?") – and the feelings soon emerge.

21. **Never criticize**. Respect their behaviour (including fighting) as their best effort at coping. You can only challenge a family to change when they feel their behaviour has been understood, accepted and affirmed as their very best effort to cope with the crisis.

22. **Be respectful of emotions**, but not over-respectful. Allow crying but don't let it block communication. Have tissues ready, but as they are handed to the person it is helpful to say "What made you cry just then?" or "Do you mind talking to me while you're crying"?

23. **Explore family assumptions**. Eg 'John is never here' might be because John is frightened he might cry and upset his Dad. Family misunderstandings are often corrected by asking each person in the meeting "How is this situation affecting you?"

24. **Reframe family criticisms** ("the blame game") which cause escalating tension. Re-interpret "negative" behaviour as positive. (eg "So when you shout at your Mum it stops her worrying about your Dad – do you always get the job of protecting people in your family?").

25. **A lot more cross-fertilization is needed** between family therapists and hospice professionals in order to define useful interventions for families around the time of a death.

FENTANYL

FENTANYL PATCH (Durogesic)

Indications	<ul><li>Severe continuous pain</li><li>eg Visceral or soft tissue cancer pain</li></ul>
Available strengths	Fentanyl Patch (mcg\hour) — Equivalent 4 hourly oral morphine 25 — 15mg 50 — 30mg 75 — 45mg 100 — 60mg 200 (two patches) — 120mg
Advantages	<ul><li>Easier compliance</li><li>Less constipating than morphine</li><li>Useful in dysphagia</li></ul>
Disadvantges	<ul><li>Less flexible dosing</li><li>Takes 12–24 hours to reach full effect</li><li>Patch allergy (rare)</li><li>Patches peeling off (use micropore tape)</li><li>High doses need a lot of patches</li></ul>
Routine use	<ul><li>Stick patch to non-hairy skin</li><li>Do not shave skin (alters absorbtion)</li><li>Change patch every 3 days</li><li>Rotate skin sites</li></ul>
Changing from morphine	<ul><li>Calculate correct patch size</li><li>Continue previous analgesia for 12 hours</li><li>Use PRN morphine for breakthrough pain</li></ul>
Side effects	<ul><li>Nausea, drowsiness, constipation May persist 24 hours after patch is removed</li><li>Fever or heating of the skin (eg heat pad) increases release</li></ul>
Morphine withdrawal effects	<ul><li>10% of patients get symptoms of morphine withdrawal when changing to fentanyl patches</li><li>Warn the patient they may occur</li><li>Diarrhoea, flu-like symptoms, yawning, colic, runny nose, shivering, anxiety and (rarely) hallucinations</li><li>Can last 2–14 days</li><li>These withdrawal symptoms respond within 30–60 minutes to 5mg oral morphine.</li></ul>

FENTANYL LOZENGES (Actiq)	
Available strengths	200,400,600,800,1200,1600mcg
Description	<ul><li>Fentanyl citrate</li><li>Lozenge on a stick ("lollipop")</li></ul>
Routine use	<ul><li>For breakthrough pain</li><li>Can be used with any other analgesics</li><li>Start with lowest dose</li><li>Rub inside the cheek for 15 minutes</li><li>Onset of analgesia within 15–30 minutes</li><li>Analgesia lasts 2–3 hours</li></ul>
Adjusting strength	<ul><li>Start with 200mcg lozenge</li><li>2 lozenges can be used together</li><li>Increase strength of lozenge until breakthrough pain is controlled</li><li>If needing more than 4 a day consider increasing dose of background analgesia</li></ul>

NOTES:

The fentanyl patch should not be started in the terminal phase (too inflexible). However, an existing patch can be left in place (and replaced every 3 days), and additional diamorphine can be given in the usual way.

A study of 19 patients with cancer who were distressed as a result of morphine toxicity and changed to fentanyl reported significantly improved well being with less drowsiness and a significant improvement in cognitive function as measured by a computer-based series of tests developed to assess dementia (McNamara P., Pall. Med. 2002; 16:42–5).

FITS

First Aid	• Protect the patient • Do not restrain or put anything in the mouth • Left lateral position (once convulsions stop) • Give rectal diazepam 10–40 mg if > 5 minutes • If no response exclude hypoglycaemia • Stay with patient until fully recovered • Explain what happened • Admit if focal signs or persistent drowsiness
Causes	• Primary brain tumours • Brain metastases • Meningeal infiltration • Metabolic • Infection • Head injury • Drug or alcohol withdrawal
Assessment	• Eye witness? • Post-ictal drowsiness? • Neurological signs • Brain scan may be indicated • Biochemistry
Phenytoin (Epanutin)	• 200–400mg nocte • Long half-life • Small dose increases can cause large rise in plasma levels, with nausea, confusion • Monitoring plasma level is important • Optimum plasma level 10–20 mg\L
Sodium valproate (Epilim)	• 200mg QID – starting dose • Increase dose gradually: 200mg\3 days • Usual dose 200–400mg QID • 2.5g\day maximum • nausea (take after food) • plasma levels not helpful
Carbamazepine (Tegretol)	• 100mg daily or BD – starting dose • Increase slowly (to 100–400mg TID) • Dizziness\blurred vision (dose-related)
Midazolam (Hypnovel)	• 10–60mg\24h SC • Prevents recurrence of fits • Useful for patients unable to swallow oral anti-convulsants
Phenobarbitone	• Added if fits difficult to control • IM: 50–200mg BD (maximum 600mg/day) • SC: 200–600mg\24h – must be a water-soluble form and does not mix with other drugs (use a second pump if necessary).

Explanation	● Teach first-aid
	● Fits secondary to brain tumours often have little effect on mental function or prognosis.
	● Driving is not allowed

NOTES:

INTERNATIONAL CLASSIFICATION OF SEIZURES

<u>Generalized</u> (involving the whole brain)
- Tonic-clonic convulsions (used to be called "Grand Mal")
- Absences (used to be called "Petit Mal" – mainly in children)
- Myoclonic (usually seen in dying patients)

<u>Partial</u> (focal, but can spread and "generalize" to involve whole brain)
- Motor – eg localized twitching (frontal), lip-smacking (temporal)
- Sensory (auras – eg tingling (parietal), smells and strong emotions (temporal)
- Complex partial, focal plus staring and inattention, usually temporal lobe

Epileptic fits (seizures, convulsions) are caused by abnormal electrical discharges in the brain.

Fits occur in about 1% of hospice patients. Mainly due to brain tumours. About 20% of patients with brain metastases and about 30% of patients with primary brain tumours have some kind of seizure. Rarely fits may be due to biochemical causes (renal failure, severe hyponatraemia). Patients with longstanding epilepsy need to continue their anti-convulsants.

Anti-convulsants can prevent seizures. Monotherapy is tried first, but a combination of two anticonvulsants may be necessary. Carbamazepine, valproate, phenytoin and lamotrigine are all effective for both generalized and partial seizures. *Levetiracetam* (*Keppra*) was licensed in 2000 for partial seizures with or without secondary generalization. It is an effective add-on therapy for partial seizures not controlled by carbamazepine or valproate, and is well tolerated with few side effects and no drug interactions. Starting dose is 500mg BD, gradually increasing to 1500mg BD.

Plasma levels of anti-convulsants may be useful if fits are difficult to control. Trough levels, taken just before dose is due, should be carbamazepine 6–12 mg\L and phenytoin 10–20 mg\L. Levels of valproate not helpful.

Steroid dose may need to be increased if fits occur or increase due to brain metastases, but anti-convulsants should also be continued.

Status epilepticus means a continuous seizure lasting longer than 5 minutes, or no recovery of consciousness between fits. This is a medical emergency. Give diazepam enema 10mg, repeated as necessary, and if this fails to control it give phenobarbitone 100–200 mg SC.

Multi-focal myoclonus with sudden involuntary movements may be unilateral or bilateral and is mainly seen in dying patients. It is exacerbated by hypoglycaemia, haloperidol, metoclopramide, and by the withdrawal of benzodiazepines. It is treated with rectal diazepam or SCI of midazolam.

FRACTURES

Neck of Femur (intracapsular)	• Do not unite • Hip prosthesis • Total hip replacement if acetabulum involved
Neck of Femur (extracapsular)	• Dynamic hip screw
Shaft of femur	• Intramedullary nail • Cement filling
Proximal humerus	• Fixation difficult • Prosthesis considered • External cast (eg Plastazote)
Mid-shaft of humerus	• Intra-medullary nail
Lower humerus	• External immobilization
Pelvis	• Fixation not possible • RT • Pain relief • No weight-bearing for 2–3 weeks till pain settles
Rib fracture	• RT • Intercostal block • Local injection • Pain settles spontaneously in 4–8 weeks
Bone metastasis from Renal cancer	• Very vascular • Embolization may be necessary pre-operatively • May be solitary site of recurrence – consider total excision

NOTES:

Most pathological fractures occur in vertebrae (collapse), femur and humerus (much less commonly in the clavicle, tibia, radius and ulna). They are most commmonly seen in cancers of the breast, bronchus, prostate and myeloma, and most (except neck of femur) will unite with callus in around 3 months whatever method of fixation. Metal and cement do not interfere with RT. RT to a large lytic lesion can increase the risk of fracture – consider prophylactic pinning.

Internal fixation, followed by RT, is the treatment of choice whenever possible to reduce pain and make nursing easier.

Lightweight plastic cast (Plastazote) with velcro fasteners is most suitable for external immobilization.

Terminal care: skin traction on the leg reduces pain on movement. A 5–10 kg weight (eg a catheter bag full of water) is adequate. Diazepam or midazolam for muscle spasm. Local injection (with a long needle) of 10ml 0.5% bupivacaine and 80mg (2ml) methylprednisolone (Depomedrone) into the fracture site can reduce pain. Dextromoramide 2.5–5mg PRN can help to reduce pain before nursing procedures.

GASTROSTOMY

Percutaneous endoscopic gastrostomy (PEG) is indicated if a patient with dysphagia develops thirst or hunger.

Insertion : The tube is inserted via endoscope under sedation and local anaesthetic. Insertion may not be possible if there is ascites, gastric ulcer, previous abdominal surgery or if the patient is on warfarin. Aspirate the tube before feeds for the first 2–3 days to detect any gastric stasis (to prevent aspiration of feed into the lungs). A tube can last 1–3 years (unless blocked or displaced). The patient can bath and shower as normal after 14 days (swimming is possible with a water-proof dressing).

Feeding can start after 12 hours, once bowel sounds are present. About 2L\day of liquid food, (eg Ensure,) is given by a battery-operated pump. The infusion is started at 50ml/hour and increased to 100ml/hour by day 3. Overnight feeding allows the patient to be disconnected from the pump during the day.

Liquid medication can be given via the tube.

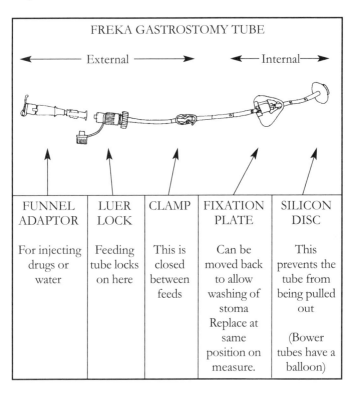

FREKA GASTROSTOMY TUBE				
← External →			← Internal →	
FUNNEL ADAPTOR	LUER LOCK	CLAMP	FIXATION PLATE	SILICON DISC
For injecting drugs or water	Feeding tube locks on here	This is closed between feeds	Can be moved back to allow washing of stoma Replace at same position on measure.	This prevents the tube from being pulled out (Bower tubes have a balloon)

Counselling from a nutritional therapist is essential if the patient or carers are to manage the tube and pump at home (feeding regime, tube flushing, daily skin care, daily mouth care, pump maintenance etc).

GASTROSTOMY

Venting gastrostomy for managing the vomiting of malignant intestinal obstruction unrelieved by drugs was first reported in 1991 (Ashby). It was developed from the minimally invasive techniques used for PEG feeding. A series (collected over some years, several before the advent of octreotide) of 51 patients who had a venting gastrostomy showed 47/51 (92%) had relief of nausea and vomiting and many had the added benefit of being able to eat a soft diet (Brooksbank, 2002). Venting gastrostomy should be considered if octreotide has failed to control distressing vomiting and is especially likely to be effective if temporary NG suction and drainage relieved the symptoms. The tube must be placed in the dependent part of the stomach and knowledge of previous surgery is essential. It is not worthwhile if prognosis is very short, only a few days.

Nasogastric tube feeding may be needed while awaiting a gastrostomy, or as a longer-term measure for some patients who do not want a gastrostomy, or where gastrostomy is not possible. The modern fine bore soft tubes are well tolerated. Insert using KY jelly and it helps if the patient sucks a small amount of crushed ice. Before starting a feed, check it is in the stomach (rather than the lung) by squirting 5–10cc of air down the tube and listen with a stethoscope for bubbling over the stomach (or aspirate and test the aspirate is acid with litmus paper, or Xray).

HORMONE THERAPY

BREAST CANCER

Tamoxifen
- 20mg OD
- Oestrogen receptor antagonist (with weak oestrogenic activity)
- For oestrogen and/or progesterone receptor-positive breast cancer
- Adjuvant therapy for new breast cancer reduces death rate by 20–30%
- Metastatic disease: 30–60% response
- Hot flushes, nausea, risk of thrombo-embolism and endometrial cancer

Anastrozole
- 1mg od
- Aromatase inhibitor – blocks conversion of androgens to oestrogens in peripheral fat
- 1st line for post-menopausal metastatic disease
- Better tolerated than tamoxifen
- Other aromatase inhibitors include letrozole, exemestane and formestane

Progesterones
- 3rd line treatment
- Medroxyprogesterone (100–500mg OD) and megestrol acetate (40–320mg OD) most commonly used
- Nausea, fluid retention and weight gain can occur

Ovarian ablation
- As effective as chemotherapy and tamoxifen in pre-menopausal
- Can be achieved by surgery (bilateral oophrectomy), radiotherapy (X-ray menopause) or medically (LHRH analogues)

NOTES:

Breast cancers that are oestrogen receptor positive respond to hormone therapy in about 50% of cases. In post-menopausal women with metastatic disease, hormonal therapy is generally preferred to chemotherapy, unless the disease is visceral and life threatening, when a rapid response to treatment is required. Clinical response to hormone therapy may take 1–3 months. Response is most likely in women over 60 with a long disease-free interval. Pre-menopausal women with metastatic disease who do not respond to initial therapy, may be offered ovarian ablation plus anastrozole.

Progesterones are also used for metastatic endometrial cancer, and produce response rates of 10–40%, with a median response of 10 months. .Progesterone receptor positive and well differentiated tumours do best.

PROSTATE CANCER

LHRH (gonadorelin) analogues

- Goserelin (Zoladex), leuprorelin (Prostap), buserelin and triptorelin
- "Medical castration" by inhibing LHRH production.
- Reduces testosterone levels by 95%
- As effective as bilateral orchidectomy
- May cause "tumour flare" due to initial transient rise in testosterone (blocked by giving anti-androgen for 2 weeks before and after starting LHRH analogue)
- SC injection (monthly or 3–monthly)
- 80% respond (median time to progression 18 months)
- Loss of libido, impotence, hot flushes, gynaecomastia, fatigue, osteoporosis, hair loss can all occur

Anti-androgens (non-steroidal)

- Flutamide and bicalutamide
- Block androgen receptors on prostatic cells
- Testosterone levels may rise (less loss of sexual potency)
- Used with LHRH analogues or as 2nd line treatment
- Bicalutamide 150 mg OD licensed for locally advanced disease
- Hot flushes, gynaecomastia, decreased libido can occur

Anti-androgens (steroidal)

- Cyproterone acetate (CPA)
- Blocks androgen receptors
- Progestogen-like action – decreases testosterone levels
- 70% respond
- Monitor LFTs (potentially hepatotoxic)
- Can be used to treat hot flushes

Stilboestrol

- Usually 2nd/3rd line treatment
- High response rates, but risk of thromboembolus
- Use in combination with aspirin
- 1–3mg OD
- Gynaecomastia, impotence, oedema and thrombosis can occur

NOTES:

For metastatic prostate cancer maximum androgen blockade (MAB) consists of LHRH analogue or bilateral orchidectomy plus a non-steroidal anti-androgen. A recent meta-analysis has shown only a 2–3% absolute 5-year survival benefit of MAB over monotherapy, so most clinicians start with monotherapy. When the disease progresses the withdrawal of anti-androgens can give a further response rates of 20% with a 4–5 month median response time. Hormone relapsed prostate cancer has a poor prognosis, with a median survival of only 6 months. (Hormone therapy also improves survival when combined with radiotherapy for localised prostate cancer.)

HYPERCALCAEMIA

Causes	<ul><li>Malignancy</li><li>Parathyroid adenoma (rare)</li><li>Tamoxifen flare</li></ul>
Assessment	<ul><li>Calcium above 2.6 mmol\l.</li><li>Measure serum PTH? (see notes)</li><li>Drowsiness</li><li>Nausea\vomiting</li><li>Large urine output</li><li>Thirst</li><li>Confusion</li><li>Dehydration</li><li>Renal failure</li><li>Is it a terminal event?</li></ul>
IV fluids	<ul><li>2–3 l saline\24 hours</li><li>Potassium supplements needed</li><li>Corrects dehydration</li><li>Only lowers calcium by 0.3 mmol\l</li></ul>
IV biphosphonates	<ul><li>eg zoledronic acid 4mg IV over 5–10 minutes</li><li>Withhold if serum creatine is above 250 micromol\l– rehydrate first</li><li>Effect takes 3–7 days</li><li>80% become normocalcaemic</li><li>Effect lasts 20–30 days</li><li>Pyrexia can occur for 24 hours</li><li>Monitor calcium weekly</li><li>Hypocalcaemia rarely occurs</li></ul>
Calcitonin (Calsynar)	<ul><li>SC 200u TID</li><li>Acts within 24 hours</li><li>Reduces calcium by about 0.5 mmol\l</li><li>Effect only lasts 2–3 days</li><li>Oral steroids prolong the effect</li><li>Nausea\vomiting\facial flushing</li></ul>
Oral Biphosphonates	<ul><li>eg Sodium clodronate (Bonefos) 1600mg nocte</li><li>Helps maintain normocalcaemia</li><li>Not always effective</li><li>NB food\milk\antacids\iron abolish absorbtion – avoid for 1 hour</li><li>Nausea can occur</li></ul>
Oral steroids (high dose)	<ul><li>Lowers calcium levels in myeloma and lymphoma</li><li>Effect is slow and partial</li><li>Little effect in most solid tumours</li><li>Increases effective of calcitonin</li></ul>
Hormones	<ul><li>Can prevent recurrence of hypercalcaemia in breast cancer</li></ul>

NOTES:

Hypercalcaemia means a calcium level above 2.6mmol\l. The typical symptoms of hypercalcamia usually only occur once the calcium level is above 2.8mmol\l. Nausea and drowsiness tend to occur first, followed by polyuria, thirst and confusion as the level rises above 3.5mmol\l. Above 4.0mmol\l death occurs in a few days if left untreated (renal failure, arrythmias, fits).

If the albumin level is low, it can make the calcium level appear low. Correct calcium level by adding 0.02mmol\l for every gram of albumin below 40g\L.

Cancer is the commonest cause of hypercalcaemia, and it occurs in about 15% of cancer patients at some stage. It is most common in cancer of the breast and myeloma. Hypercalcaemia is also associated with squamous cancers, eg lung, oesophagus, head and neck, renal, cervix and ovary and with the haematological malignancies: lymphomas and leukaemias. It rarely occurs in small cell lung cancer and with adenocarcinomas, eg prostate, gastric, colon. Prostate cancer with extensive bone metastases still rarely causes hypercalcaemia.

The mechanism of hypercalcaemia in malignancy is a protein secreted by the tumour that ressembes PTH (parathyroid hormone) which reduces calcium excretion in the distal convoluted tubule. Bone metastases tend to worsen it by releasing more calcium into the blood stream. In myeloma and lymphoma there are also osteoclast-activating factors. The high level of calcium suppresses normal PTH, so assay of PTH shows low levels in cancer (because the tumour-secreted protein that ressembes PTH is not measured).

Measure PTH if hypercalcaemia is the only sign of a suspected recurrence of cancer, as it may be due to a benign parathyroid adenoma, when PTH will be high.

Prognosis tends to be poor once hypercalcaemia has occurred: 80% survive less than one year.

Zoledronic acid has superseded other bisphosphonates. It is a third generation bisphosphonate that is more potent than pamidromate in inhibiting bone resorbtion. It has a longer duration of action (5 weeks versus 3 weeks) and a higher response rate (90% compared to 70%). 4mg IV is given every 4-6 weeks. If there is no response try 8mg (about 50% respond for a median of 2 weeks). Transient fever occurs within 48 hours in 30%, and nausea may occur.

IV saline, 1L every 6 hours with potassium supplements should be given if dehydrated or if the level is above 3.5mmol\l. Saline alone will only reduce calcium levels by 0.2–04mmol\l.

Calcitonin is rarely needed, but has the advantage of a faster onset of action than the biphosphonates. Calcium levels begin to fall after 2 hours. It is sometimes used if calcium levels are very high or if symptoms are severe. The effect lasts 2–3 days, but is prolonged to 6–9 days by high dose steroids. It tends to worsen nausea – give anti-emetics

Steroids have a poor response rate, and are no longer used routinely, but they can boost the effect of calcitonin and still have a place in lymphomas and myeloma.

Octreotide has been used to treat hypercalcaemia in neuro-endocrine tumours.

INSOMNIA

Assessment	• Bedtime, time of getting to sleep, waking times?
	• What is their normal pattern?
	• Worrying?
	• Fear of dying in sleep?
	• Environment? (noise, heat, light)
	• Relaxing bedtime routine?
	• Sleeping pills tried?
	• Ask their partner's opinion
	• Day-time naps?
	• Coffee, alcohol, fluid intake?
	• Symptoms at night?
	• Mattress comfortable?
	• Bedclothes\pillows?
	• Preferred positioning?
	• Nightmares?
Treat symptoms causing insomnia	• Anxiety\depression
	• Pain\stiffness
	• Wheeze or cough
	• Itch
	• Cramps
	• Sweating
	• Frequency or incontinence
	• Steroids – insomnia
Use short-acting hypnotics	• Titrate to a full dose
	• Tolerance after 2–3 weeks (use intermittently)
Treat depression	• Early waking suggest depression
	• Amitriptyline 50–150mg ON is sedating
Treat anxiety	• Lorazepam 1mg BD or diazepam 5–10mg OD
	• Haloperidol 5mg ON if agitated
	• Chlorpromazine 25–50mg ON for extra sedation
	• Counselling\Relaxation\Massage
Quinine	• Prevents night cramps
	• 200mg or 300mg ON
	• Usually effective
Desmopressin	• Reduces nocturnal frequency
	• 100–300mcg ON
	• Use tablets (not nasal spray)
Relaxation	• Massage\aromatherapy
	• Night light
	• Relaxation tapes

NOTES:

Sleep deprivation is used as a form of torture. Poor sleep is very distressing and makes the control of all symptoms more difficult. Take inability to sleep very seriously.

Short acting hypnotics such as zopiclone 7.5–15mg or temazepam 10–60mg can bring a lot of relief. Titrate to a full dose before deciding it does not work. Intermittent use prevents tolerance (develops over 3–14 days of continuous use).

Avoid long-acting drugs, like nitrazepam and flunitrazepam, which cause "hangover" drowsiness.

SLEEPING PILLS

	Median half-life (in hours)
Zolpidem (Stilnoct) 5–10mg	2
Chlormethiazole (Heminevrin) 1–2 caps	4
Zopiclone (Zimovane) 3.75–7.5mg	5
Chloral (Welldorm) 1–5 tablets	8
Temazepam 10–60mg	13
Nitrazepam (Mogadon) 5–10mg	30
Flunitrazepam (Rohypnol) 0.5–2mg	30

Chlormethiazole (Heminevrin) capsule (192mg) or syrup (250mg in 5ml) is useful short term in the elderly, as it is short-acting and has no hangover effect, but it is addictive if used continuously.

Ask about dreams or nightmares in detail, not to attempt analysis but to allow the verbalization of fears. Nightmares may be due to denial, which may need gently challenging.

Fear of dying while sleeping is common (hearing "you will die peacefully in your sleep" may be a factor). Explanation can help.

Severe insomnia can be overcome with an IM injection of a combination of diamorphine 2.5mg, levomepromazine 50mg and hyoscine hydrobromide 0.4mg – this lasts about 4 hours.

The function of sleep remains unknown, but it is essential for life. Animals deprived of sleep eventually die. Sleep is currently thought to rebalance neurotransmitters, re-model synapses and process the day's emotions.

INTESTINAL OBSTRUCTION

Diagnosis	<ul><li>Abdominal distension</li><li>Colic</li><li>Vomiting</li><li>Constipation (no motions or wind)</li><li>AXR – fluid levels</li></ul>
Palliative colostomy	<ul><li>Seek a surgical opinion if there is the possibility of a single, correctable block in a relatively fit patient.</li></ul>
Subcutaneous Infusion of Drugs	<ul><li>Diamorphine (for aching pain)</li><li>Buscopan 60mg\24h (for colic) Cyclizine 150mg\24h (for nausea)</li></ul> [Diamorphine dose = 50% of 24 hour oral morphine]
Dexamethasone	<ul><li>6–12mg\24h</li><li>Can resolve pyloric obstruction</li><li><u>May</u> increase the chance of lower obstruction resolving</li></ul>
Octreotide (Sandostatin)	<ul><li>100mcg BD by SC injection</li><li>300–600 mcg\24h SC</li><li>Reduces GI secretions</li><li>Reduces volume of vomits</li><li>In one study of 24 patients with vomiting from malignant obstruction, 14 had no further vomiting (Riley 1992)</li></ul>
Lactulose	<ul><li>10–20ml BD</li><li>Softens motions</li><li>Milpar 10ml BD is an alternative</li><li>Bowel function can return</li><li>Avoid stimulant laxatives (colic)</li></ul>
Loperamide	<ul><li>2–4mg QID</li><li>Controls diarrhoea</li><li>Diarrhoea can be a feature of malignant bowel dysfunction.</li></ul>
NG aspiration	<ul><li>For distressing vomiting that is not controlled by octreotide.</li></ul>
Venting Gastrostomy	<ul><li>Alternative to NG tube for persistent distressing vomiting</li><li>Allows oral feeding</li><li>See Gastrostomy</li></ul>

INTESTINAL OBSTRUCTION

IV fluids	• Indicated if the patient is thirsty (unusual) • 2–3L\24 hours • Patients with obstruction can still absorb oral fluids above the level of the block and usually remain well hydrated.
Explanation	• Abdominal swelling is due to bowel distension, not to spreading cancer. • A diagram can be helpful • The aim: control pain and abolish nausea • Occasional vomiting may be inevitable • Eating and drinking is possible • Soft diet and fluids encouraged • Laxatives (softeners) still given

NOTES:

Malignant obstruction of the bowel may present suddenly with pain and vomiting or it may come on gradually over weeks or months. The pattern can vary as the disease progresses. It may gradually worsen or become continuous or sometimes may resolve and become intermittent. The mechanism can be occlusion of the gut lumen, or extramural compression, or malignant adhesions, or motility disorders due to tumour infiltration of intestinal muscle or mesentery, and it can occur at several sites. *Abdominal distension* is most pronounced with obstruction of the colon but may be minimal with small bowel obstruction (especially with a lot of adhesions) and is absent with duodenal obstruction (large volume vomits with no colic). Malignant bowel dysfunction is often a more accurate concept than obstruction, because diarrhoea can occur as well as constipation, and bowel function can return again, sometimes after many days of obstruction.

Incidence: 3% of patients with far-advanced cancer, most commonly due to ovarian and large bowel cancers, but occasionally other cancers (pancreas, endometrium, cervix).

The medical management of intestinal obstruction was first described in 1985 (Baines et al) and can relieve the symptoms of obstruction and enable the patient to drink and eat. Until then, patients with advanced cancer who obstructed were sent for surgery, and\or managed with IV fluids and NG suction which does not relieve the symptoms of pain, colic, nausea and vomiting. *Venting gastrostomy* for severe vomiting in malignant intestinal obstruction unrelieved by drugs was first reported in 1991 (See Gastrostomy). The somatostatin analogue *octreotide* (*Sandostatin*) has been used since 1992 to relieve obstructive vomiting and to reduce the diarrhoea caused by subacute obstruction. Abdominal pain, colic and distension are also improved and side effects are minimal. *Steroids* (dexamethasone 8–12mg\day) are used in obstructed patients to reduce peri-tumour oedema and open up the obstruction. Small studies have reported benefit but there have been no randomised trials.

See: Gastrostomy, Subcutaneous infusions.

ITCH

Assessment
- General or localised ?
- Biliary obstruction?
- Drug-induced? (opioids, aspirin, amphetamines, phenothiazines)
- Medical? (Renal failure, diabetes, iron deficiency)
- Haematological? (lymphoma, leukaemia, polycythaemia)
- Skin condition? (urticaria, folliculitis, pemphigoid)
- Fungal allergy?
- Infestation? (lice, scabies, fleas)
- Paraneoplastic? (breast, colon, lung, stomach)
- Consider referral to dermatologist\skin biopsy

General measures
- Treat dry skin
- Avoid alcohol and spicy foods
- Avoid heat (hot baths, strong sunlight, vasodilators)
- Avoid rough clothes
- Electric fan to cool skin
- Keep nails short, cotton gloves at night
- Avoid dehydration, anxiety and boredom

Emollients
- Rehydrate dry skin
- Dry skin worsens all types of itch
- Aqueous Cream BP
- Oilatum 15ml per bath
- Use as a soap substitute

Biliary stent
- Treatment of choice for obstructive jaundice
- Alternatives are surgical bypass (cholecystjejunostomy), external bile drainage (percutanous transhepatic route by interventional radiology) RT to nodes at porta hepatis or high-dose steroids.
- Ureteric stent for obstructive renal failure

Creams and lotions for itching

● 2.5% Hydrocortisone	–	Eczema due to scratching
● Calamine lotion	–	Cools by evaporation
● Menthol 2%	–	Chilling sensation
● Capsaicin cream	–	Depletes Substance P (Initial burning)

NB Crotamiton is not effective

Stanozolol
- 10mg OD. Anabolic steroid.
- Can reduce itch in obstructive jaundice (discovered 1951)
- Mechanism unknown
- May deepen jaundice
- Withdrawn March 2001 (danazol now tried)

Anti-histamines
- Non-sedating eg Loratadine 5mg OD for urticaria or allergy
- H2 antagonists eg ranitidine 150mg BD can reduce paraneoplastic itch

Night Sedation
- Hypnotics (see Insomnia)
- Sedating anti-histamine, eg chlorpheniramine 4–8mg ON
- Amitriptyline 50–100mg ON (known anti-pruritic action)
- Doxepin 75mg ON ((known anti-pruritic action)

5HT3 antagonists
- e.g ondansetron
- Proven effective for uraemic, opioid-induced and cholestatic itch
- Use traditional antiemetic doses

Other approaches (occasionally tried)
- Cholestipol 10mg BD (in partial biliary obstruction)
- SSRI (for paraneoplastic itch)
- NSAID (if cutaneous malignancy itches)
- Rifampicin, naltrexone (for cholestasis)
- Danazol instead of stanozolol
- Thalidomide
- UVB phototherapy (for mobile patients)
- Behavioural treatment
- Hypnotherapy
- Transcutaneous electronic nerve stimulation (TENS)
- Acupuncture
- Plasma exchange

NOTES:

Itch (pruritus) is related to pain (and can be equally distressing). It is mediated by C-fibres like pain, but itch receptors are more superficial that pain receptors. They are triggered by histamine, prostaglandins, bile acids or tissue proteinases. Itch is made worse by skin vasodilation (heat, alcohol, spices, drugs such as nitrates) anxiety or boredom. It can also be caused centrally, eg by a brain tumour. Pathogenesis is complex and not fully understood, and as yet there are no generally effective anti-pruritic drugs. Itch can also cause excoriation, secondary infection, insomnia and depression.

In severe itching the first step in management is to ensure a good night's sleep.

LISTENING SKILLS

Preparation
- Calm down (eg meditate for a few minutes)
- Make some "inner space"
- Give your own concerns some listening time
- Finish doing anything urgent
- Consider time boundaries

Concentration
- Look at the person
- Remember what they say!
- Notice body language
- Do not interrupt
- Tolerate long pauses

Self control
- Be aware of your own emotions
- Keep your opinions to yourself
- Stay calm, don't over-react to ideas\words

Encouragement
- Non-verbal (nods, smiles)
- Seek more information ("Is there anything else?")
- Be sensitive "It seems difficult for you to talk about this."

Responding
- Be relevant
- Use open questions ("What, Why, How?")
- Focus on the answer (not your clever question)
- Do not talk about yourself

Reflective questions
- Eg responding to "How long have I got?" with
  "What makes you ask me that right now?" or
  "Is that something you have been worrying about?"
- Encourages talking
- Avoids wrong assumptions, premature explanation\opinion
- Keeps the focus on the person

Tracking
- Notice key words, and turn into a question ("Your
  daughter?")
- Most effective with non-sequiturs (linked to unconscious)
- Always leads to relevant further discussion

Repeating
- Draws the speaker's attention to what was said
- A way of emphasing ("Your husband finds it difficult")

Clarifying
- Ensures you understand what is being said
- Eg "Can you explain again about ...."
- Also a way of exploring ("Are you saying....?")

Clarifying (continued)
- USEFUL QUESTION: "What assumptions might you be making about that?"

Linking
- You said "A" and earlier "B" – is there a connection
- Link up reported events, experiences, reactions, ideas
- Can result in new insights

Using silence
- Allows time for person to listen to their own words
- Notice that their eyes move as they "see" new connections
- Needs to be friendly and relaxed
- Ask "What were you thinking about?"

Noticing discrepancies
- Eg "You just said …, BUT earlier you seemed to be saying…"
- Can lead to fresh insights for the person
- Trust is needed first

Verbalizing empathy
- Attempted understanding of other's situation
- "It seems that you are feeling….."
- Be tentative, you may be wrong
- Very therapeutic for the other person

Summarizing
- KEY skill – can be repeated several times
- "So what I think I am hearing you say is …"
- Summarize what you heard (NOT your opinions of it!)

Ending
- Be affirming (eg "You have been very honest")
- Be aware of the priviledge (eg "Thank you for sharing")

NOTES:

Active listening is one-way, whereas social listening is two-way. Active listening takes energy and is tiring.

The aim is to provide a space for the other person to listen to themselves ("How do I know what I feel, until I hear what I say?").

Listening skills need to become second nature, so you don't start to think *about* the skills, and stop listening (once the TV is tuned in, we turn our attention to the show). Practice them with a colleague – one skill at a time (eg "What is your main concern at the moment?").

You are not listening when:	
* You are in a hurry	* You change the subject
* You think about yourself	* You assume you know what I'm going to say
* You interrupt	
* You ask the same question twice	* You over-react to certain words
* You don't ask any questions	* You feel critical of me

LYMPHOEDEMA

Assessment	• Swollen limb (gradual onset) • Non-pitting oedema • Lymphatic damage • Hard skin • "Elephant skin" • No response to diuretics
Compression bandaging (multi-layered)	• Used for severe or hard lymphoedema or lymphorrhoea • Elastic bandage is used (eg Secure Forte). • Re-applied daily for 2 weeks • Repeat every 6–8 weeks • Velband first to protect the skin • Stop if fluid-shift causes pain
Compression pump	• Speeds up initial compression • Not superior to bandaging • Keep pressure below 60 mm Hg
Elastic support garments	• Predetermined pressure • Increase lymphatic drainage • Limb movement helps • Worn all day • Removed at night

Massage (manual lymph drainage)	• Stimulates lymph flow in the superficial lymph vessels
	• Can shift lymphoedema from
	  • head and neck
	  • trunk
	  • genitalia.
	• Gentle milking action moves lymph in skin lymphatics
	• Start in <u>healthy</u> area and work towards oedema.

Exercises	• Active or passive • Reduces swelling by increasing lymph flow • Should be done with elastic support
Skin care	• Regular aqueous cream (skin hydration) • Use work gloves • Avoid: cuts\scratches\pressure\heat\detergents • Scaling – Calmurid cream
Antibiotics	• eg flucloxacillin 500mg QID • Infection can be sub-clinical • Suspect if worsening swelling or malaise • Repeated infections worsen lymphoedema

Antibiotics (continued)	• Consider prophylactic antibiotics • NSAID for repeated inflammatory episodes not responding to antibiotics
Paroven	• 1g TID • Decreases venous permeability and lymph formation • May soften lymphoedema • Takes months!
Heavy arm	• Collar and cuff for walking (avoid a sling – elbow stiffens). • Support flat when sitting • Gentle bandaging (for support not compression) can increase comfort • Low dose morphine for ache • NB Elevation not effective

NOTES:

Lymphatic vessels contain interstitial fluid, and flow is increased by limb movements and skin massage. The larger vessels are contractile and have valves.

Lymphoedema is swelling of the subcutaneous tissues due to damaged lymphatics (due to surgery, RT or malignant infiltration). It is high-protein oedema. Blocked lymphatics initially causes pitting oedema, but in time fibrin and fat are deposited and swelling becomes irreversible and non-pitting ('brawny'). Skin fibrosis and hyperkeratosis occurs and the skin becomes susceptible to infection and cellulitis.

The aim of treatment in advanced cancer is often simply to minimize further swelling and to improve comfort. Treatment with massage and compression therapy can be time-consuming and the burden of treatment must not outweigh the benefits. In bedbound patients gentle passive movements can reduce stiffness and discomfort.

Elastic stockings available on prescription are a lower compression class (<40mm Hg) than the garments needed for lymphoedema, which must be obtained via a surgical appliance department or bought privately. Shaped tubigrip (single or double layer) is a useful alternative for some situations and easier to apply.

Treatment is in 2 phases. A Reduction phase (compression bandaging and massage) and a Maintenance phase (elastic hosiery). Both phases include exercises and skin care. Compression bandaging and massage, performed correctly, can reduce even long-standing swelling from lymphoedema.

Steroids are usually ineffective, but can occasionally reverse early lymphoedema (eg dexamethasone 4–8mg daily).

Diuretics are usually ineffective, but sometimes there is an element of venous obstruction and some pitting oedema superimposed which may reduce partially with diuretics.

Hiccups	• May be due to gastric distension, liver metastases, mediastinal nodes (pressure on phrenic nerve) or uraemia.
	• Asilone 10–20ml PRN
	• Metoclopramide 10–20mg TID
	• Lioresal (Baclofen) 5–30mg TID
	• Nebulized saline
	• Nifedipine 20mg TID (may lower BP)
	• Haloperidol 1–5mg
	• High dose steroids
	• IV chlorpromazine 25–50mg (slowly)
	• SC midazolam 100–200mg\24h (sedating)
Hoarse voice	• Laryngeal nerve palsy
	• Laryngeal thrush (rare)
	• Teflon injection (refer for ENT opinion)
	• Ketoconazole suspension
Muscle Spasms	• Baclofen (Lioresal) 5–30mg TID
	• Tizanidine (Zanaflex) 2mg OD
	• Dantrolene (Dantrium) 25–100mg TID
	• Quinine sulphate, 200mg for cramps
	• Diazepam (Valium) 2–10mg at night
Smell	• Metronidazole 200–400mg TID
	• Metronidazole gel topically
	• Electric air filter
	• Wound cleaning\remove slough
	• Charcoal dressings
Tremor	• Exaggerated physiological tremor
	• Anxiety
	• Alcohol
	• Thyrotoxicosis
	• Drug-induced (eg salbutamol)
	• Familial
	• Parkinsonism (at rest)
	• Cerebellar damage (intention tremor)

NOTES:

Hiccups are due to muscle spasms (diaphragm and intercostals) causing a sudden inspiration that is terminated by closure of the epiglottis over the larynx. They occur separately to the respiratory reflex and have negligible effect on ventilation. Rate can be 4–60 per minute. Persistent hiccups (>48 hours) are commoner in men (4:1). They can cause exhaustion and insomnia, can exacerbate pain and cause social embarrassment. There is no universal remedy (one patient who hiccupped for 8 years received 60,000 letters suggesting possible cures!). Traditional remedies include pharyngeal stimulation, swallowing ice, breath-holding or breathing into a paper bag (raising pCO2), or bending forward. Nebulized saline can be very effective. Chlorpromazine was described as effective in 1955. Lioresal (Baclofen), a muscle relaxant, is the treatment of choice because it has been proven to be effective by a randomised controlled trial. Nifedipine has the advantage of causing no drowsiness but can lower BP. Phrenic nerve compression may respond to high dose steroids. Phrenic nerve block abolishes the diaphragmatic spasms but not the intercostals spasms.

Hoarse voice is usually due to recurrent laryngeal nerve palsy usually secondary to a left hilar tumour. It starts suddenly and is painless. The patient can be reassured that the voice will not disappear altogether. Teflon injection pushes the paralysed cord medially, so that it opposes with the functioning cord. This can restore the voice to normal. Laryngeal thrush is a rarer cause of hoarseness, usually associated with inhaled steroids. It can be difficult to eradicate.

Muscle spasms occur in MND and in spastic paraplegia due to cord damage. Drug doses need to be balanced so that the spasms are reduced without causing floppiness. Baclofen and tizanidine acts at the spinal level, whereas dantrolene acts peripherally, and they can be used together. Diazepam (Valium) 2–10mg at night, can be useful for night spasms. Quinine sulphate, 200mg or 300mg at night can reduce night cramps.

Smell may be due to cutaneous malignancy (fungation), lung abscess causing foul halitosis, or a necrotic rectal tumour causing a smelly discharge. Smell can be reduced within 2–3 days by oral metronidazole (Flagyl) 400mg TID, and then maintainance treatment, 200mg TID, is then necessary. It may cause nausea and can cause severe headaches with alcohol. Longterm use may (rarely) cause a neuropathy. Chloramphenicol 500mg QID, will also reduce smell due to anaerobes, and has a place for patients who cannot tolerate metronidazole. Metronidazole gel (Metrotop) applied daily to fungating skin tumours is soothing and controls smell very effectively in 90% of patients, but is expensive. Deodorant sprays are best avoided, as they mix with the smell rather than removing it. An electric air filter makes life more bearable for patient and carers.

Tremor from any cause is worsened by anxiety. Exclude thyrotoxicosis and consider trying propranolol 20–40mg QID (contra-indicated with asthma). Nebulized ipratropium (Atrovent) causes less tremor than nebulized salbutamol (Ventolin).

MORPHINE 1 – Usage

Indications
- Severe continuous pain
- Some pains respond poorly or partially eg neuropathic

Routine use
- Oral route is most effective
- Start with 2.5–5mg 4 hourly
- Liquid (Oramorph) or tablet (Sevredol)
- Increase the dose every 4 hours, till painfree
- Usual increments: 2.5, 5, 10, 20, 30, 60, 90 mg 4 hourly
- No maximum dose
- Start laxative day 1 – eg codanthramer 10ml BD.
- Patient needs access to rescue dose for 'breakthrough' pain (= regular dose in mg)

Modified release
- Useful for maintainance treatment
- First calculate 24 hour dose of morphine (regular+rescue)
- 12 hourly eg MST, Zomorph, Oramorph SR
- 24 hourly eg MXL, Morcap SR
- All are equi-analgesic
- eg Oramorph 30mg 4h = MST 90mg BD = MXL 180mg daily
- 4 hourly still needed in case of breakthrough pain

Adjusting the dose
- Pain breaking through – increase dose
- Painfree and drowsy – reduce the dose
- After a nerve block – reduce the dose
- Drowsy, still in pain – other measures needed

Side effects
- Constipation
- Drowsiness
- Nausea (occurs for first 48h in 30%)
- Dry mouth
- Blocked ears (5%)
- Sweats (rare)
- Itch (with spinal morphine)
- Constricted pupils

Drowsiness
- Is it distressing?
- Is it due to morphine?
- Reduce dose if painfree
- Consider opioid switch? (fentanyl, oxycodone)
- Consider adding methylphenidate 5mg BD
- Consider spinal morphine

Drug interactions
- Rare
- Avoid MAOIs (hypertensive crisis, agitation)
- Alcohol is safe when on regular morphine

The morphine myths
- Extensive clinical experience now documented
- Fears of addiction, sedation and respiratory depression are unfounded
- Can be safely continued for many months.
- If the pain is controlled by a different method (e.g. a nerve block), morphine can be stopped without difficulty, ie addiction is not a problem when it is used for pain.

SC injection
- Useful if unable to take morphine orally
- Peak plasma concentrations within 20 minutes
- Less painful than IM
- Conversion from oral to SC – divide by 3
- Diamorphine used in UK – more soluble

Spinal morphine
- Delivers high dose to spinal receptors
- Indicated for side effects or partial response
- Epidural dose = 10% of 24h oral dose
- Intrathecal dose = 1% of 24h oral dose
- Addition of bupivacaine may improve pain control

Intravenous morphine
- May be preferred (rarely) if:
  - indwelling IV line
  - Generalised oedema
  - SCI problems (erythema, sterile abscesses)
  - Coagulation disorders
  - Poor peripheral circulation
  - Conversion from oral to IV – divide by 3

Other routes
- Rectal – safe and effective (equi-analgesic with oral)
- Buccal, sublingual, nebulised – not recommended (absorption unpredictable)

NOTES:

A routine checklist is very helpful when monitoring a patient on morphine. Ask regularly about:

A = Anxieties about using morphine?
B = Breakthrough pain?
C = Constipation?
D = Drowsiness?

Driving is safe in alert patients on a stable dose. A stable dose of morphine has been shown to have minimal effects on cognition.

Active metabolites may contribute to toxicity, particularly in patients with renal impairment.

MORPHINE 2 – Formulations

Morphine preparations	Strengths	Notes
Oramorph solution (4 hourly)	10mg\5ml – clear 100mg\5ml – pink Oral vials 10, 30, 100mg – all 5 mls	
Sevredol tablets (4 hourly)	10mg – blue 20mg – pink 50mg – green	Tablets are scored and easily halved
MST Continus Tablets (12 hourly)	5mg – white 10mg – brown 15mg – green 30mg – purple 60mg – orange 100mg – grey 200mg – green	Effective rectally Some patients need TID (rarely)
MST Continus Suspension (12 hourly)	20mg 30mg 60mg 100mg 200mg	All sachets contain pink granules
Zomorph capsules (12 hourly)	10mg – yellow\clear 30mg – pink\clear 60mg – orange\clear 100mg – white\clear 200mg – clear\clear	Contain pellets that can be sprinkled on food or given via a gastrostomy tube
Oramorph SR Tablets (12 hourly)	10mg – brown 30mg – purple 60mg – orange 100mg – grey	Same colour code as MST
Morcap SR Capsules (24 hours)	20mg – clear + 2 stripes 50mg – clear + 3 stripes 100mg – clear + 4 stripes	Contain pellets that can be sprinkled on food or given via a gastrostomy tube
MXL Capsules (24 hours)	30mg – light blue 60mg – brown 90mg – pink 120mg – green 150mg – dark blue 200mg – red-brown	

MORPHINE 2 – Formulations

NOTES:

Start with 4 hourly preparations and once pain control is achieved on a steady dose, change to a modified release preparation.

The modified release formulations of morphine (tablets, capsules or liquids) are all similar in their duration of effect and relative analgesic potency.

The time to reach peak plasma levels following a single dose is faster for the normal-release forms of morphine (1 hour) compared to the 12 hour modified-release preparations (2.7 hours) or the once daily preparations (8.5 hours), but with repeat dosing this is not clinically important.

MOUTH PROBLEMS

Routine Mouthcare	<ul><li>Foam stick after meals</li><li>Regular toothbrushing</li><li>Soak dentures</li><li>Vaseline\Nivea to dry lips</li><li>Flavoured lip gels</li><li>Nystatin 1ml QID if on steroids\antibiotics</li><li>Mouthwash (see below)</li></ul>
Dry Mouth	<ul><li>Rehydrate if thirsty</li><li>Drug-induced?</li><li>Thrush?</li><li>Routine mouth care 1–2 hourly</li><li>Crushed ice</li><li>Glandosane spray (plain or lemon)</li><li>Saliva Orthana spray</li><li>Pilocarpine</li></ul>
Coated Tongue	<ul><li>Effervescent vitamin C tablet on tongue TID</li><li>Miconazole (Daktarin) gel</li><li>Pineapple slices</li><li>Bocasan mouthwash</li><li>Soft toothbrush</li></ul>
Thrush	<ul><li>Nystatin 1ml QID</li><li>Ketoconazole 200mg BD</li><li>Fluconzole 50mg daily</li></ul>
Apthous ulceration	<ul><li>Triamcinolone paste (Adcortyl in orobase)</li><li>Carbenoxolone</li><li>Bioral gel</li><li>Bioplex mouthwash QID</li><li>Choline salycilate gel (Bonjela)</li><li>2.5% hydrocortisone pellets (Corlan)</li><li>Benzocaine (Dequacaine) lozenges</li><li>Tetracycline mouthwash (see notes)</li></ul>
Soreness	<ul><li>Re-line dentures?</li><li>Rinse with soluble aspirin</li><li>Benzydamine mouthwash</li><li>Benzydamine spray</li><li>5% lignocaine paste</li><li>Gelclair</li></ul>

NOTES:

Gelclair is a gel that coats the mouth and can reduce oral pain from ulceration or malignant invasion. It is used as a rinse (not swallowed) TID before meals, 15ml in each sachet either diluted with 20–40ml of water, or used undiluted for severe pain. It is not a drug, and is not absorbed, but coats the oral mucosa and forms a protective barrier. It contains polyvinyl-pyrrolidone and sodium hyaluronate. It tastes of aniseed (which some patients dislike).

Herpetic ulceration in AIDS can be severe and is treated (or prevented) with oral acyclovir (Zovirax) 400mg 5 times a day, plus locally applied cream.

Tetracycline mouthwash is used for recurrent aphthous ulceration. The contents of 250mg capsule in small amount of water, held in mouth for 2 minutes, TID. It predisposes to oral thrush.

Pilocarpine 5mg TID (tablets) stimulates saliva (and increases the mucin in saliva so it is more protective). It can be useful for treating a dry mouth but unfortunately it also causes sweating, which puts many patients off. Diarrhoea, nausea and flushing can occur. In one study half the patients preferred it to artificial saliva. It acts on the parasympathetic system. Maximum effect may take 4–8 weeks. Maximum dose 10mg TID. It cannot work if there is no salivary function.

0.2% chlorhexidine (Corsodyl) is very active against the organisms in dental plaque and reduces halitosis (but causes reversible brown staining of teeth).

Thalidomide 100mg daily is a very effective treatment for severe apthous ulceration. It is used in HIV disease but side-effects are common (headache, drowsiness, constipation); named-patient basis only.

NAUSEA AND VOMITING

Assessment	<li>**History**<ul><li>Drug-related?</li><li>Recent RT\chemo?</li><li>Headaches (raised ICP)?</li><li>Situational (anxiety)?</li><li>Large volume (pyloric stenosis)?</li><li>Dyspepsia\reflux – try metoclopramide</li><li>Movement related – try cyclizine</li><li>Thirst\drowsiness (hypercalcaemia)?</li><li>Dysuria (UTI)?</li><li>Constipation?</li></ul><li>**Examination**<ul><li>Papilloedema\neurological signs</li><li>Abdomen and PR</li></ul><li>**Tests**<ul><li>MSU</li><li>U&E, calcium</li><li>CXR (?RTI)</li></ul>
Treat Reversible Causes	<ul><li>Drugs – Stop\change</li><li>Anxiety – Anxiolytics</li><li>Brain Metastases – Steroids</li><li>Gastritis – Ranitidine</li><li>Cough – Anti-tussives</li><li>Constipation – Laxatives</li><li>UTI or RTI – Antibiotics</li><li>Hypercalcaemia – IV biphosphonate</li></ul>
Consider Surgery	<ul><li>Gastro-jejunostomy for duodenal obstruction (eg CA pancreas)</li><li>Palliative colostomy for low intestinal obstruction</li></ul>
Oral anti-emetics	<ul><li>For <u>prevention</u> of nausea</li><li>eg prochlorperazine 5mg TID</li><li>eg haloperidol 1.5mg nocte</li><li>NB established nausea causes gastric stasis and prevents oral absorption</li></ul>
IM anti-emetics	<ul><li><u>To settle an episode</u> of nausea</li><li>eg prochlorperazine 12.5mg</li><li>eg cyclizine 50mg</li></ul>
Anti-emetic Suppositories	<ul><li>For established nausea\vomiting</li><li>eg prochlorperazine 50mg TID</li><li>eg cyclizine 50mg TID</li><li>eg domperidone 30–60mg TID</li><li>eg chlorpromazine 100mg nocte</li></ul>
SC infusion of anti-emetics	<ul><li>For established nausea\vomiting</li></ul> Usual starting dose Cyclizine 150mg\24h Metoclopramide 60mg\24h Haloperidol 5mg\24h Levomepromazine 6.25mg\24h

Combination of anti-emetics	• 25% need two anti-emetics to control nausea and vomiting • eg SC infusion of cyclizine with halperidol
Add steroids?	• SC Dexamethasone 8–12 mg\24hr • Anti-emetic action • Potentiates other anti-emetics • Can relieve malignant pyloric obstruction (large volume vomiting) in about 50% • Precipitates with cyclizine and levomepromazine (consider separate infusion)
Levomepro-mazine	• SC 6.25 mg\24h • Powerful anti-emetic but sedating. • Broad spectrum anti-emetic
Ondansetron	• IV 32mg then oral 8mg BD, or • SC 20mg\24h • Mainly to prevent cytotoxic-vomiting • Can work for other causes (GI or CNS) when other drugs fail • Acts at 5HT3 receptors • Expensive
Octreotide	• SC 200–600 micrograms\24h • Reduces G.I. secretions and motility • Can reduce volume of vomit in intestinal obstruction
Nasogastric Aspiration or Venting gastrostomy	• If large volume vomits are distressing and not controlled by octreotide • See Gastrostomy
I.V. Fluids	• Consider if dehydrated, especially if thirst occurs.
Remember Anxiety	• Vomiting can be frightening (am I dying?) • Fear can worsen vomiting • Consider anxiolytics • Family counselling?

NOTES:

The commonest mistakes are persisting for too long with the oral route for anti-emetics (nausea causes gastric stasis) and not considering reversible factors. Anti-emetics need to be given systemically first to gain control. Stopping subcutaneous infusions of anti-emetics is often possible once nausea and vomiting have settled, BUT start oral anti-emetics before stopping SC infusion.

See also Anti-emetics, Intestinal obstruction, Subcutaneous drugs, Subcutaneous infusions.

NERVE BLOCKS

Coeliac Plexus	• Upper abdominal pain: (eg cancer of pancreas, stomach, liver)
	• 80% get relief
	• Effect lasts 12 months
	• Postural hypotension occurs for 24h
	• Diarrhoea can occur for 24h
	• Complications (rare):
	  • retroperitoneal haematoma
	  • L1 neuritis
	  • kidney puncture

Paravertebral Thoracic	• Chest wall pain • Vertebral metastases • Oesophageal pain (T3–5) • Covers several dermatomes • 5ml aqueous phenol • Can be repeated • Complications are rare
Intrathecal Neurolytic	• Perineal pain (L5\S1) in already bedbound, catheterized patient • Unilateral trunk pain • Risk of leg weakness\urinary incontinence
Intercostal	• Rib metastases or fractures • Cryoprobe\radio-coagulation
Brachial plexus	• (supraclavicular, interscalene or axillary) • Arm pain – usually nerve pain in an already paralysed arm • Note: use continuous infusion of bupivacaine before a neurolytic block, because some patients prefer pain to numbness
Sacral	• Buttock pain • Sacro-iliac block via sacral hiatus
Epidural steroids	• Vertebral body pain
Hip block	• Acetabular metastases • Femoral head metastases
Trigeminal	• Facial pain
Bilateral lumbar sympathetic	• Tenesmus • Pelvic visceral pain (rectum, bladder, uterus) • Superior hypogastric plexus block may be more effective

NOTES:

Nerve blocks are considered when other methods of pain control are not effective, and are usually performed by an anaesthetist with a special interest in Pain Clinic work.

Stop warfarin before blocks.

Change modified-release formulations of morphine to 4–hourly morphine prior to the block, in case the pain is abolished.

Stop morphine temporarily after the procedure (to avoid respiratory depression if the block has abolished the pain). If pain recurs give 5mg morphine and increase the dose step by step in the usual way until painfree. Ask regularly about pain for the first 1–2 days.

NSAIDS

CLASSIFICATION OF NSAIDS

NON-SELECTIVE COX-INHIBITORS

Proprionates
- Ibuprofen 400mg TID
- Naproxen 250–500mg BD

Acetates
- Diclofenac 50mg TID
- Indomethacin 25–50mg QID

PREFERENTIAL COX-2 INHIBITORS
- Meloxicam (Mobic) 7.5–15mg daily
- Etodolac (Lodine SR) 600mg daily

SELECTIVE COX-2 INHIBITORS
- Celecoxib (Celebrex) 100–200mg BD
- Rofecoxib (Vioxx) 12.5–25mg daily
- Fewer GI side effects (70% fewer ulcers, 40% fewer symptoms of dyspepsia)

Uses of NSAIDs (in palliative care)
- Painful bone metastases
- Headache
- Sweating
- Skin pain
- Bladder spasms

Routine use
- Do not use more than one NSAID at a time
- Do not use with low-dose aspirin (GI bleed more common)
- Start with lowest recommended dose
- Consider changing to a different type if effect is poor (40% respond better to one NSAID than another)
- Consider changing if side effects occur (main differences between NSAIDs is in incidence and types of side effects)

Mode of action
- Anti-inflammatory (full effect takes 3 weeks)
- Analgesic (as effective as morphine 5mg IM for some pains)
- Inhibition of cyclo-oxygenase (COX) enzymes needed for prostaglandin synthesis from arachidonic acid.
- The non-selective NSAIDs block COX-1, which produces normal prostaglandins needed for gastric mucosa integrity and platelet and renal function (hence their side-effects) as well as blocking COX-2 enzymes which mediate pain and inflammation.
- Preferential NSAIDs inhibit COX-2, more than COX-1, but still inhibit COX-1

Contra-indications
- Active peptic ulcer (use high dose PPI such as lanzoprazole first, to heal the uler)
- Allergy to any NSAID or aspirin

Side effects of NSAIDs
- Side effects are more common and more severe in the elderly
- GI upset, dizziness and drowsiness are the commonest side effects.
- Worsening of asthma can occur with any NSAID
- Reduced platelet function can occur with the non-selective NSAIDs, so avoid them with chemotherapy or thrombocytopenia
- Renal effects include fluid retention, raised BP, worsening renal function or rarely haematuria, papillary necrosis or renal failure
- Other side effects include diarrhoea, nausea, rashes, wheeze, headache (and rarely hepatic damage and alveolitis)

Gastric side effects
- GI side effects are least common with celecoxib and rofecoxib, low with ibuprofen, moderate with diclofenac, naproxen, ketoprofen, piroxicam and meloxicam, and highest with aspirin and azapropazone.
- GI side effects can occur even when NSAIDs are given rectally or IM
- 25% of chronic NSAID users will develop peptic ulceration (most commonly gastric) but 50% of them have no symptoms.
- 20% of chronic users will develop symptoms of dyspepsia but 50% of them will have no evidence of peptic ulceration on gastroscopy.
- If at risk of peptic ulceration use selective NSAIDs and/or give gastro-protection with omeprazol 20mg, which is significantly more effective than ranitidine. Misoprostol is as effective as omeprazole but causes diarrhoea in 40% and is therefore rarely used.

NOTES:

NSAIDs are most commonly used in palliative care for relief of pain from bone metastases while awaiting radiotherapy or while waiting for it to take effect.

They are given orally where possible. If patients are not able to take tablets, suppositories (eg diclofenac 100mg or ketoprofen 100mg) are useful. The IM route relieves pain faster than the oral route, and SC infusions (eg diclofenac 150mg per 24 hours) can relieve severe bone pain that is not relieved by oral NSAIDs.

OEDEMA

Assessment	• Bilateral swelling (soft) of ankles • Pitting on sustained pressure
Causes	• NSAIDs\steroids? (fluid retention) • Heart failure? • Dependent oedema? (immobility) • Low serum albumin?
Improve mobility	• Calf muscles act as pump • Walking reduces ankle oedema • Passive leg exercises help
Elevation of legs	• legs must be above horizontal • Support whole of limb
Support stockings	• Above knee • Stop if uncomfortable
Bendrofluazide	• 5–10mg daily • Only a mild diuretic
Frusemide	• 40–80mg daily • Diuresis within 1 hour (lasts 6 hours) • High doses needed in renal failure • Avoid at night (diuresis disturbs sleep) • Hypotension can occur • Hypokalaemia can occur
Amiloride	• 5–10mg daily • Potassium-sparing • Given with frusemide to prevent hypokalaemia
Spironolactone	• 100–200mg daily • Given with frusemide • Potassium-sparing • Nausea • Gynaecomastia
Metolozone	• 5–20mg daily • Potent diuretic • Combine with frusemide • Useful for resistant oedema
Compression Pump	• Shifts soft oedema very rapidly • Beware precipitating heart failure by sudden shift of fluid • Keep pressure below 60 mm Hg • Follow with support stockings
IV Albumin	• Short-lived effect • Only raises plasma albumin for 1–2 days • Rarely appropriate

NOTES:

NB Stop diuretics if diuresis is more troublesome than the ankle swelling.

For severe oedema consider a temporary indwelling urinary catheter and high dose diuretics BD.

Unilateral leg oedema suggests lymphatic obstruction from pelvic tumour (see Lymphoedema) or a DVT (see Thrombosis).

Bilateral leg swelling may be due to IVC thrombosis

Swelling of the ARM may be due to:

- lymphoedema   - unilateral
- SVCO   - bilateral
- Axillary vein thrombosis   - unilateral

PAIN 1 – ASSESSMENT

Assessment is based on the patient's verbal report. It is important because continuous pains (visceral and soft tissue) respond to morphine, whereas other pains (bone, nerve, colic, or non-cancer pains eg migraine, angina) need other approaches.

ASSESSMENT OF PAIN

DESCRIPTION	TYPE	TREATMENT
"Continuous"	Visceral or Soft tissue	Morphine
"On movement"	Bone	RT NSAIDs Biphosphonates Exclude fracture
"Stabbing" "Burning"	Nerve	Morphine Tricyclics Anti-convulsants Steroids
"Comes and goes"	Colic	Buscopan
On breathing	Pleuritic	
Episodes of pain	Gastric distension Bladder spasms Tenesmus Ureteric	See Pain Syndromes
Atypical pattern	? infection ? central	

The routine approach to pain control = MANAGE

M : Morphine
A : Adjuvant drugs (Co-analgesics)
N : Nerve blocks
A : Anxiety or Depression?
G : Go back to oncologists?
E : Emotional\family issues?

(See Pain Treatments)

A BODY CHART is useful for <u>initial assessment</u>, because it serves as a communications tool by making the pain "visible". It demonstrates the sites of pains (80% have two or more pains) and makes a record for the notes. It should be drawn with (or by) the patient.

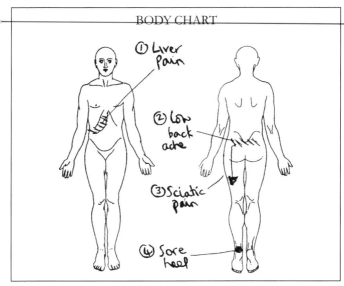

BODY CHART

PAIN SCORES are a simple way to monitor difficult pain control. The patient is asked 3 times a day to rate the severity of pain on a score of 0–10, where 0 is no pain at all and 10 is the worst pain imaginable. The scores are recorded on a chart, or kept as a diary. They are useful to monitor responses to different treatments and allow early changes in therapy.

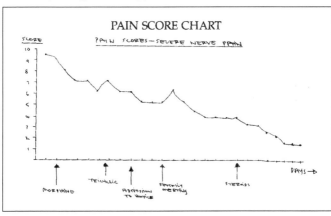

PAIN SCORE CHART

PAIN 2 – SYNDROMES

Visceral\Soft tissue pain (continuous pain)	• Opioids • Nerve blocks (needed by 5% of patients)
Bone pain	• Radiotherapy (80% respond) • NSAIDs • Morphine if severe or continous • Biphosphonates (not proven)

Nerve pain	• Opioids (partial response)
	• Imipramine 25–150mg, with
	• Anticonvulsant:
	  • Carbamazepine 100–200 mg TID
	  • Sodium valproate 200–400mg QID
	  • Phenytoin 200–300mg nocte
	• Flecainide 100mg BD (stop tricyclic)
	• Trial of steroids
	• Spinal morphine
	• Nerve blocks
	• Cordotomy

Colic	• Buscopan 10–20mg QID orally or SC 60–120mg\24h • Octreotide 200–600 mcg\24h SC
Liver Pain	• Opioids • Steroids • Coeliac plexus block • Embolization (rarely)
Pressure sores	• Benzydamine (Difflam) cream beneath occlusive dressing • Oral NSAID
Headaches	• Tension – paracetamol • Skull metastases – bone RT • Raised ICP – steroids\brain RT • Diclofenac 150mg\24h by SC infusion if severe (unusual) • Opioids if very severe (rare)
Pleuritic pain (on inspiration)	• NSAID or RT (rib pain) • Antibiotics (infection) • Anti-coagulate for PE • Intra-pleural bupivacaine (if severe)
Gastric distension Pain	• Antacids • Metoclopramide 10–20mg TID
Head and Neck Tumours	• Opioids • Steroids • Broad spectrum antibiotics • Trigeminal block

Scar Pain	<ul><li>? Stitch (remove)</li><li>? Neuroma (excise)</li><li>Local nerve block</li><li>Tricyclic\anticonvulsant</li></ul>
Painful Procedures (eg dressings)	<ul><li>Dextromoramide (see Analgesics)</li><li>Entonox</li><li>Nebulised fentanil?</li><li>IV midazolam (reversible with IV flumazenil)</li></ul>
Tenesmus	<ul><li>Painful sensation of wanting to open the bowel</li><li>Exclude impacted faeces</li><li>Low dose morphine</li><li>NSAID suppositories</li><li>RT to shrink?</li><li>Transanal resection\cryo\laser to debulk?</li><li>Steroid enema (colifoam) BD</li><li>Bupivacaine enema</li><li>Lumbar sympathetic block</li></ul>
Bladder Spasms	<ul><li>Exclude infection</li><li>Low dose morphine</li><li>Oxybutinin 5mg TID</li><li>Buscopan (high dose)</li><li>Lumbar sympathetic block</li><li>0.25% bupivacaine bladder washouts</li></ul>
Ureteric pain	<ul><li>SC Diclofenac</li><li>Buscopan</li><li>Steroids</li><li>Ureteric stent</li></ul>
Pelvic Pain	<ul><li>Opioids</li><li>Steroids</li><li>Antibiotics</li><li>Spinal morphine</li><li>Intrathecal phenol (perineal pain)</li><li>Epidural bupivacaine for severe pain if patient already bedbound and catheterized.</li></ul>
Herpes zoster (Shingles)	<ul><li>Acyclovir</li><li>Tricyclic</li><li>Anticonvulsant</li><li>Capsaicin cream</li></ul>
Thalamic Pain (central pain)	<ul><li>Unilateral burning pain in arm and leg</li><li>Amitriptyline, with chlorpromazine</li></ul>

PAIN 3 – TREATMENTS

Opioids	• Very effective for visceral or soft tissue pain (ie continuous pain) • Increase dose every 4 hours till pain controlled. (See Morphine) • Start laxative!
Radiotherapy	• Treatment of choice for bone pain • 80% get relief in 1–2 weeks • Low dose (palliative) RT has few side effects.
NSAIDs	• eg Naproxen 500mg BD • Effective for bone pain • 20% get gastritis • SC diclofenac may control difficult pains
Tricyclics	• Indicated for any pain that is only partially controlled by morphine (usually nerve pain). • eg imipramine 25–50mg BD • known analgesic action • Act via monoamine pain modulating pathway
Anti-convulsants	• For nerve pain (burning, stabbing) • Gabapentin, valproate, carbamazepine • Stabilize nerve membrane (?) • eg Phenytoin 300mg nocte • eg Sodium Valporate 200–400 QID • Can use <u>with</u> tricyclics.
High dose steroids	• eg dexamethasone 6–12 mg\day • Reduces peri-neural oedema • Reverses early nerve compression
Buscopan	• 10–20mg TID or 60–120mg\24h SC • Relieves colic in malignant intestinal obstruction
Antibiotics	• Pain from head and neck tumours that stops responding to morphine may be due to cellulitis and can respond to broad-spectrum antibiotic.
Other Co-analgesics	• NSAIDs – Bone pain • Biphosphonates – Bone pain • Anxiolytics – Anxiety • Anti-depressants – Depression • Baclofen – Spasms • Quinine – Night cramps • Oxybutinin – Bladder spasms • Steroid enemas – Tenesmus • NSAID suppositories – Tenesmus

Spinal morphine	• "Spinal" = epidural or intrathecal • For pain not controlled by above measures or if morphine drowsiness is distressing (see Morphine).
Nerve Blocks	• For pain not responding to the above measures (see Nerve blocks)
Chemotherapy	• Can reduce pain by shrinking tumour, especially in breast cancer, head and neck tumours and sarcomas.
Local methods of pain relief	• TENS\Acupuncture • Skin traction • Heat pad • Inject trigger point with local anaesthetic
Emotional Support (essential overcome difficult pains)	• Raises pain threshold • to Ensure quality sleep • Counselling (patient and family) • Relaxation therapy • Massage • Creative activities • Short-term goals • Religious support
Embolization (rarely)	• Most useful to control renal pain from kidney tumours
Ketamine (rarely)	• Specialist use for difficult pains • 100–300mg\24h by SC infusion • Can be effective orally 20–100mg daily (In one study 3 out of 21 had a good response) • Sedating – reduce morphine • Hallucination can occur (not dose-related) • Acts at spinal N-Methyl-D-Aspartate receptors • Contra-indicated in epilepsy
Cordotomy (very rarely)	• C1\C2 (mastoid level) • Indication: severe unilateral pain below C5 not controlled by above measures • 80% get pain relief (contralateral side) • Numbness and tingling can be unpleasant • Ipselateral leg weakness can occur. • Relief lasts 1–2 years. • Patient must be able to co-operate during the procedure

PAIN 4 – Patient Information

People with cancer pain often have unnecessary fears based on a number of myths.

Myth 1: The cancer will cause terrible pain at some stage.

30% of people with cancer never get any cancer pains. If you do get pain the majority of cancer pains (85%) can be easily controlled, provided you tell somebody about them.

Myth 2: My pain will get worse and worse as my cancer progresses.

Firstly, your pain may not be due to cancer, but something else. Secondly, cancer pain does not necessarily get worse even if the cancer progresses. Thirdly, most cancer pains remain well controlled right up to the time of death.

Myth 3: If I admit to having pain it means I am giving in and I will lose the respect of my doctors and nurses.

Communicating about your pain is not complaining it is enabling the doctors and nurses do their job, which is to control your pain. Your pain is invisible, so you need to describe it and work in partnership with your professional carers, in order to control it.

Myth 4: If I mention pain the doctors may assume the cancer has spread and give up on my treatment.

Pain can occur at any stage in cancer and does not mean that treatments such as radiotherapy or chemotherapy will be stopped, as these can also help control pain.

Myth 5: If I take painkillers now they won't work later when I really need them.

This is the fear of needing higher and higher doses to keep the pain controlled. The technical term for this is "drug tolerance". This does NOT occur with morphine or other strong pain medicines when they are used to control pain.

Myth 6: Once you start on morphine it means the beginning of the end.

Morphine is a simple painkiller, which is particularly effective for constant aching pains. It has no effect on your lifespan and some patients with non-malignant pain such as arthritis stay on the same dose of morphine for many years.

Myth 7: If my pain does not respond to morphine it means my disease is out of control.

Some cancer pains respond well to morphine but some do not and then other approaches are needed. An episode of severe pain does not mean that your life will be shortened by it.

Myth 8: If I start morphine I will get addicted to it.

It is impossible to get addicted to oral morphine that is used for pain. If you start taking regular morphine you can safely stop it at any time. Your pain would probably return, just as before, but you would NOT get any of the effects of addiction such as sweats, cramps or craving for it, because you would not be addicted, even if you had been on it for a long time.

Myth 9: Morphine will make me a "zombie" and sleep all the time.

If you are painfree on morphine but feeling drowsy that means the dose of morphine needs reducing. Make sure you report any drowsiness to your doctor or nurse. The main side effect of strong painkillers is constipation.

Myth 10: If I start morphine I may not be allowed to continue with my other complementary therapies.

Morphine will not interfere with any of your other treatments and in fact morphine has very few interactions with other drugs. Anything that improves your pain control will be encouraged.

Myth 11: If I keep taking painkillers I won't know if the pain goes away?

If you have constant pain it is best to take regular painkillers ("by the clock") to control it. Stopping the painkillers will only make the pain come back. Having pain saps your energy. Keeping the pain controlled releases some of your energy for other activities.

PERICARIAL EFFUSIONS

Assessment	<ul><li>Dyspnoea\chest discomfort</li><li>Hypotension, tachycardia, absent apex beat</li><li>JVP rises on inspiration</li><li>CXR shows enlarged heart</li><li>ECG shows low voltage, elevated ST segments</li><li>Prognosis can still be in months</li></ul>
Aspiration	<ul><li>Performed under echocardiogram</li><li>Relieves symptoms</li><li>Instillation of cytotoxics is not helpful</li></ul>
Radiotherapy	<ul><li>Can prevent recurrence</li><li>Not if previous RT to chest</li><li>Not if previous doxorubicin</li></ul>
Pericardial surgery	<ul><li>Subxiphoid pericardiotomy (10% mortality)</li><li>Pericardial window via thoracotomy (65% mortality)</li></ul>
Balloon Pericardiotomy	<ul><li>Percutaneous, under local anaesthetic</li><li>Indicated for recurrent effusion</li><li>Safe and effective</li><li>Can cause a pleural effusion</li></ul>

NOTES:

Median survival with a pericardial effusion is 3–4 months with non-small cell lung cancer and around 9 months with breast cancer. Many are not detected.

Assessment	• Dyspnoea, cough and pleuritic pains • Absent breath sounds • Dullness to percussion • Chest Xray shows basal opacity • Lateral decubitus Xray or ultrasound confirm fluid rather than pleural thickening
Pleural aspiration	• Lateral chest • Sixth intercostal space • On top of rib (to avoid the neurovascular bundle) • 1–1.5L is drained • Aspirate under ultrasound if loculated • Stop if coughing or dizziness (mediastinal shift) • Avoid in terminal hours
Bleomycin	• 60iu (40iu in the frail and elderly) • in 100cc of saline plus 20ml 1% lignocaine • Instilled after effusion is drained • IV hydrocortisone 100mg reduces fever\pain • Prevents recurrence for one month in 70%
Talc pleuradesis or Pleurectomy	• Considered for recurrent effusion in a patient with a prognosis of months. Both performed under GA • Effective for around 90% of cases • Refer to thoracic surgeon

NOTES:

Most malignant effusions are from breast or bronchus. The pleura is unusual as a single site of relapse, and usually an expression of metastatic disease elsewhere. Survival can still be over 2 years in breast cancer. Not all effusions are malignant (eg heart failure). No treatment is needed if it is symptomless. Simple aspiration is usually the best option, repeated as necessary. The main risk of aspiration is a pneumothorax, which can often be managed by simple aspiration of the air rather than a chest drain and underwater seal. For recurrent effusions a sclerosing agent can be inserted, but the effusion should be drained to dryness first. Tetracycline and bleomycin are the most effective agents. Tetracycline causes pain ("like scalding water") when instilled and therefore bleomycin is preferred.

PRESCRIBING

CHECKLIST	COMMENTS
Review current medication	• Examine <u>all</u> medicines being taken • Ask how each is taken • Ask who is in charge, patient or carer?
Drug History	• Previous drugs tried/abandoned? • N.B. analgesic history • N.B. steroid history
Allergies	• Ask for full details of "allergic reactions"
Preferences\Attitudes	• eg tablets or liquids • Beliefs about drugs • Complementary treatments
Making drug changes	• Include patient in decision-making • One change at a time is best • Explain reasons • Follow up on effects • Can a drug be reduced\stopped?
Prescribing a New Drug	• Any contra-indications? Allergies? • Any interactions? • Check dose • Explain purpose • Mention side-effects • Remember PLACEBO EFFECT

PLACEBO effect	• Patients benefit more from any drug if they believe it will be effective.
	• This effect can last weeks or months
	• It depends on:
	  – Doctor's enthusiasm when prescribing
	  – Patient's trust
	  – Patient's role in decision making

Consider Route	• Oral\sublingual\Buccal • Transdermal patches • Inhaled • SC infusion • Rectal suppository • IM/SC injection • IV (rarely)
Vomiting	• Vomiting of oral drugs – repeat dose? • Oral drugs are absorbed after 1 hour
Compliance	• Use a DRUG CARD • Explain to patient and carer • Consider pre-loaded pill dispenser? • Follow up

Plasma levels	• Can be important in the use of some drugs (eg digoxin, phenytoin, theophyllines).
Emotional aspects of prescribing	• Patients often blame drugs rather than illness • Doctors can hide behind prescribing – it is easier to prescribe than listen. • Inappropriate focus on drugs can waste valuable opportunities for patient to adjust emotionally

NOTES:

A drug card lists medication, times they are taken (often 9 1 5 9) and purpose of each drug. A drug card plus explanation greatly improves understanding of drugs and effectiveness of symptom control. Find out who is in charge of the medicines.

EXAMPLE DRUG CARD

TIMES: DATE:

Tablets/Medicines	9	1	5	9	(1)	(5)	Purpose
	AM	PM			AM		
MST 30mg	1			1			Regular Pain Control
Co-proxamol	2	2	2	2	(2)	(2)	Extra Pain Control
Metoclopramide 10mg	1	1	1	1			To prevent nausea
Dexamethasone 2mg	2						Appetite
Co-danthramer	10ml			10ml			Bowels
Temazepam 10mg			bed-time 1				Sleep

See also Drug interactions

PRESSURE SORES

Cause	<ul><li>Ischaemic skin damage</li><li>Pressure above capillary pressure (25mm Hg) for 1–2 hours</li><li>Bony prominences increase pressure</li><li>Note – normal pressure over the ischial tuberosities when sitting is 300mm Hg!</li></ul>
Risk factors	<ul><li>Assessed by various scores (eg Waterlow)</li><li>Factors that increase the risk are:<ul><li>Low weight</li><li>Thin, oedematous or broken skin</li><li>Age</li><li>Poor mobility</li><li>Incontinence</li><li>Poor appetite</li></ul></li><li>SPECIAL HIGH RISKS are: cachexia, heart failure, diabetes, paraplegia, peripheral vascular disease, steroids</li></ul>
Vulnerable pressure points	<ul><li>Sacrum (sitting, lying)</li><li>Hips, elbows, ears, shoulders (lying on side)</li><li>Thoracic spine (if thin and kyphotic)</li><li>Heels (lying in bed)</li></ul>
Prevention	<ul><li>Educate</li><li>Improve mobility</li><li>Pressure-relieving mattress</li><li>Chair cushion\heel pads</li></ul>
Treatment	<ul><li>Relieve pressure, improve mobility</li><li>Reduce friction damage (skilled lifting\turning)</li><li>Moist wound healing (modern dressing)</li><li>Remove slough (delays healing)</li><li>Surgical debridement, larval therapy</li><li>Skin grafting</li></ul>

CLASSIFICATION OF PRESSURE SORES

	Healing time (if pressure relieved)	Possible Dressing
1 Blanching redness	2 hours	–
2 Persistent redness	2 days	Semi-permeable
3 Ulcer	1–2 weeks	Hydrocolloid
4 Ulcer + Exudate	3–4 weeks	Hydrogel, foam
5 Cavity	Months	Alginate ribbon

NOTES:

A pressure sore is tissue damage caused by unrelieved pressure and capillary compression. It only takes 1-2 hours of pressure above 25mm Hg to block capillary flow and cause irreversible tissue damage.

Prevention of pressure sores involves having (and using) an effective policy of risk assessment, selection of appropriate support surfaces, skin care with regular use of emollients, improving mobility if possible, moving and handling strategies and regular re-assessment of risk.

Risk Assessment tools for pressure sores (Waterlow, Norton, Braden) all consider the main risk factors, which include mobility, weight, age, sensory loss, friction\shear, nutrition, hydration, continence and skin moisture, or special high risk factors (see opposite).

Pressure relieving equipment includes heel and elbow pads, soft mattress covers, air-wave mattresses or specialized beds with air sacs or micro-spheres that 'suspend' the patient and reduce pressure enough to allow healing even if immobile.

Healing occurs if pressure is relieved. Any wound heals better with warmth and moisture, and modern dressings promote moist wound healing. Wounds do not have to be sterile to heal, and strong antiseptics should be avoided as they damage fibroblasts and delay granulation. Slough should be removed as it predisposes to infection and slows healing because it contains proteolytic enzymes (see Wound Healing).

QUESTIONS

QUESTIONS ABOUT SYMPTOMS
- What has worried you most about this symptom?
- Which of your symptoms is giving you the most trouble?
- If it weren't for the pain, how would you be feeling?
- Have you known anyone else with cancer?
- What problems do\did they have?
- How do you feel about me changing your treatment?

QUESTIONS ABOUT ILLNESS
- What has been the most difficult part of this illness for you?
- How has this illness affected your life\your family\your children\your relationship together?
- What do you do to keep your spirits up?
- What would you be doing now if you were suddenly well again?
- How did you feel about coming into the hospital/hospice.

QUESTIONS ABOUT FEELINGS
- Have you known anyone else with cancer?
- Do you feel frightened at times? What about?
- What has been the worst part of this illness?
- What is the worst thing that could happen?
- When do you feel frightened?
- Do you mind talking while you cry?
- What made you cry just now?

QUESTIONS ABOUT PROGNOSIS
- What have you been told about your illness?
- How do you see the future?
- How long are you hoping for?
- If the time comes for you to need more nursing help, (or to die) where would you like to be looked after? Why?

QUESTIONS ABOUT INSIGHT
- How do you feel things are going at the moment?
- What do you understand about your illness?
- How did you feel when the doctor told you about it?
- Do you ever feel it may be more serious?
- What does your family feel about your illness?
- Do you think it might help you to know more about your illness?

NOTES:

Interlace questions about symptoms with questions about feelings, ie ask about feelings EARLY in an assessment interview (eg "How did you feel about that?"). This increases the accuracy of <u>all</u> the information received, and enables patients to disclose other important concerns. It does not have to be time-consuming, and it increases both patient and professional satisfaction.

Open questions (What, Why, How?) tend to open up communication and encourage the patient to talk about feelings.

Closed questions (Do you, Have you, Are you?) tend to close down conversation, by encouraging a yes or no answer, but can be useful to clarify specific points.

Leading questions invite a particular reply (eg "Are you <u>all right</u> today?" instead of "How are you feeling today?"), and indicate a lack of willingness to listen.

Reflective questions are a very useful when asked difficult questions (eg the response to the question "How long have I got?" might be: "Is that something you have been thinking about?"). It avoids giving inappropriate information. If you are uncertain what to say, ask a question about what the patient just said.

Hypothetical questions starting with IF are very useful to explore attitudes to the future (eg "IF you need more help in the future, would you want to stay at home or be admitted..?") and can also give a fresh perspective on emotions such as guilt (eg "IF this illness had happened to your partner, how would you have felt then?").

Techniques that increase a patient's ability to disclose concerns include open questions, summarizing the concerns, checking ("Do you want to talk more about...?"), making educated guesses about feelings and clarifying (eg "What exactly do you mean by devastated?"). Avoid closed questions, leading questions, multiple questions (asking several things at once) and premature advice or premature reassurance.

NB Always ask questions <u>before</u> giving information, explanation or advice. The aim of asking questions is to find out about the patient's concerns.

RADIOTHERAPY (Palliative)

Bone pain
- 60–80% respond
- May respond in 2–3 days, maximum effect after 2–4 weeks
- Single dose 8 Gy as effective as fractionated course
- Short courses (20Gy in 5 fractions) for pathological fractures, spinal cord compression
- Speeds healing of pathological fractures
- Widespread bone pain treated with hemi-body RT or strontium 89
- Hemi-body irradiation is safe and effective. A single fraction is given to upper body (6Gy) or lower body (8Gy). Pain relief in 80%. Give anti-emetics. Check Hb
- Strontium 89 injection is as effective as external RT. Can repeat if blood counts OK.

Spinal cord compression
- 8% of cancer patients
- RT emergency – immediate steroids, same day RT
- Short course is standard treatment – eg 20 Gy in 5 fractions
- Allow patient to mobilise early if pain free
- 80% of patients who can walk at start of treatment will remain ambulatory
- Only 5% of paraplegic patients regain walking after RT

Brain metastases
- *Steroids* – 8–16mg dose. 70% respond
- *Radiotherapy* for multiple metastases in relatively fit patient with no active metastases elsewhere. 50% get improved symptoms (eg weakness), median survival 2–7 months
- *Neurosurgery* considered for solitary metastases. Median survival 12 months
- *Chemotherapy* may be preferred for small cell lung cancer, lymphomas and breast cancer
- Non-small cell lung cancer – brain RT unlikely to be of benefit
- Common RT schedule is 12Gy in 2 fractions. 30Gy in 10 fractions if good prognosis
- Hair loss occurs, but it re-grows. Headaches and nausea occur occasionally. Somnolence syndrome can occur 2–10 weeks later

SVC obstruction (see p. 146)

Lung cancer
- Haemoptysis (90% get relief)
- Chest pain, SOB, cough (50% get relief)
- Useful for compression of bronchus causing lung collapse
- Short treatment schedules are effective e.g 17 Gy in 2 fractions

RADIOTHERAPY (Palliative)

Other uses of palliative RT
- Control bleeding (lung, bladder, rectum, vagina)
- Unblock hollow organ (bronchus, oesophagus)
- Cranial nerve lesions due to skull base metastases
- Choroidal metastases (60–70% benefit)
- Leptomeningeal disease
- Splenomegaly
- Pelvic malignancy
- Lymphadenopathy if painful/bulky/ulcerating

Side effects of RT (depends on dose, fractionation and site)
- Skin reaction (see below)
- Malaise, fatigue (with high doses)
- Nausea, diarrhoea (pelvis/abdomen)
- Reversible hair loss (brain)
- Cystitis (bladder)
- Oesophagitis (mediastinum)
- Mucositis (head and neck)
- Somnolence syndrome (brain)
- Pneumonitis (chest)
- Lhermitte's sign – electric shock like pains with neck flexion (spinal cord)

Skin reaction
- Redness and soreness
- Starts 1–2 weeks after first treatment
- Can last 3 weeks after last treatment
- Avoid wetting\shaving\sunlight\perfumed soaps
- 1% hydrocortisone cream if sore
- Pigmentation fades after 1 year

NOTES:

50% of all cancer patients will require radiotherapy at some point during their illness and around half of these treatments are palliative.

Radical radiotherapy (high dose) aims for cure or local tumour control. It is given to the limits of normal tissue tolerance.

Palliative radiotherapy (usually lower dose) aims to relieve/prevent symptoms, improving quality of life and possibly extend survival, with fewer side effects. A treatment goal should be established and communicated to the patient. Patients can be confused by their palliative treatment ("If the doctors knew I had cancer cells in my body, why didn't they treat me sooner?"). Explain the aim is control not cure.

NB Variations in dose and fractionation vary widely between radiotherapists, especially in the palliative setting.

RARE PROBLEMS

Diabetes Insipidus	• Associated with hypothalamic or pituitary metastases • Can occur rarely in primary brain tumours • Lack of ADH • Large volumes of dilute urine (4–10L\day) • Thirst – onset can be sudden • Frequency disturbs sleep • Diagnosis confirmed by plasma and urine osmolality • Treated with desmopressin (DDAVP) • 100–200 mcg orally nocte or BD, or • 1–4 mcg IM nocte or BD • A single dose lasts 12 hours • Adjust dose, aim for at least 500ml of urine per day (to prevent water intoxication)
Hypoglycaemia	• Associated with retroperitoneal tumours and hepatoma (rare) • Blood glucose below 2.2 mmol\l • Early morning stupor/shakiness • Frequent snacks • Patient should carry oral glucose • Oral steroids elevate glucose • Night feeding • Glucagon 10mg IM • IV glucose 10–50% (continuous if severe)
Ectopic ACTH	• Associated with small cell lung cancer, and rarely other tumours • Severe weakness • Hypokalaemic alkalosis • Elevated ACTH • Treat with metyrapone or aminoglutethamide • Replacement steroids

Syndrome of Inappropriate ADH (SIADH)	• Associated with small cell lung cancer (5%)
	• Drowsiness\confusion\siezures
	• Hyponatraemia (serum sodium below 125mmol\l)
	• Plasma osmolality less than 270 mOsm\kg
	• Urine osmolality over twice that of plasma
	   • Treatment:
	   • Water restriction (500ml per day)
	   • Demeclocycline (Ledermycin) 300mg QID

Gynaecomastia	<ul><li>Breast development in men</li><li>Can be painful</li><li>Usually due to castration</li><li>Can be due to drugs (spironolactone, metoclopramide)</li><li>Treatment options:<ul><li>Topical dihydrotestosterone</li><li>Tamoxifen</li><li>Liposuction</li><li>Subcutaneous mastectomy</li></ul></li></ul>

NOTES:

Thyrotoxicosis can occur rarely due to TSH-like peptides. It has been described in choriocarcinoma, testicular, breast and lung cancers and mesothelioma.

Octreotide can offer effective palliation for some rare hormone-secreting tumours. Carcinoid tumours (5HT causes wheezing, flushing and diarrhoea), gastrinoma of the pancreas (peptic ulceration), vasoactive intestinal peptide-secreting tumours ("VIP-oma") (severe diarrhoea, flushing) and insulin-secreting tumours (spontaneous hypoglycaemia).

REHABILITATION

Step-by-step Approach	1	Personal care (washing\feeding\toileting)
	2	Sitting out of bed
	3	Dressing
	4	Walking with support
	5	Walking with a frame\stick
	6	Climbing steps
	7	Assessment of daily living
	8	Home assessment (OT)
	9	Home visit
	10	Trial period at home
	11	Home with extra support
	12	Day care
	13	Booked respite admission
Prostheses	●	Wig
	●	Breast
	●	Limb
	●	Facial
	●	Liaise with specialist team
Has the patient adopted the "sick-role" too early?	●	Nurses may need to plan graded <u>reduction</u> in help
What is preventing independence?	●	Weakness
	●	Pain
	●	Dyspnoea
	●	Lymphoedema
	●	Loss of confidence
	●	Fears about future care
Are the goals appropriate?	●	Small improvements in independence are encouraging, but unrealistic goals destroy morale
What is the aim?	●	Self-caring?
	●	Wheelchair life?
	●	Partial dependence?
	●	Improved morale?
Would a wheelchair increase mobility?	●	Can be a dreaded option
	●	Wide range of wheelchairs
	●	OT assessment first
	●	Counselling

NOTES:

Rehabilitation is often resisted until confidence has been restored. A step-by-step programme enables progress to occur without the patient becoming anxious about how they will cope.

Staff must communicate together and aim for the same goals. A programme of rehabilitation is important because patients often have limited energy and can only manage to do so much each day.

Adjustment is often needed to becoming more independent again – this may take time, explanation and negotiation.

The physiotherapist can plan graded exercise programmes for specific problems, assess for appropriate equipment and can teach patient and relatives best methods for transfering, walking, use of stick or frame and climbing steps. If there are stairs in the home and the bed is still upstairs climbing steps may be the limiting factor in getting home.

The Occupational Therapist (OT) can assess the patient's ability to cope with activities of daily living (ADL) and the suitability or adaptability of the home.

SKIN PROBLEMS (General)

Dry skin	• Common problem • Use E45 cream, or • Aqueous cream as a soap substitute
Drug reaction	• Redness, weals, itch • Facial oedema • Stop new drugs • Piriton 4–8 mg TID • IV hydrocortisone if severe
Hyperkeratosis (thick scales)	• Seen in longstanding oedema • Calmurid HC cream daily – rehydrates skin
Herpes zoster (Shingles)	• Skin pain can proceed rash by 1–2 days • Small fragile blisters • Dermatome distributions with central cut-off line. • Acyclovir 800MG 4 hourly
Blistering rash	• Take swabs (? Staph) • Avoid steroids until infection is excluded. • Flucloxacillin 500mg QID • Topical mupirocin (Bactroban) • Dermatology opinion (? Pemphigus, ? drug reaction) • Consider skin biopsy

Fungation (cutaneous malignant infiltration)	• RT or chemotherapy? • Surgery/skin graft? • Cryotherapy? • Control bleeding (see Bleeding) • Control smell (see below) • pain control (morphine, NSAID) • Regular dressings (eg irrigate, metronidazole gel, paraffin tulle, gamgee padding, tubivest)
Fistulas	• Colostomy bag (to collect discharge) • Barrier cream (to protect skin) • Metronidazole (to reduce smell) • Octreotide (see intestinal obstruction) • Bypass surgery? • Facial plug (see notes)
Smell	• Metronidazole gel (held in place by paraffin tulle if necessary) • Metronidazole PO 200–400 mgQID (effective within 2–3 days) • Chloramphenical 500 mg QID also effective • Charcoal dressings • Electric air filter
Facial hair Growth (rare)	• Hypertrichosis lanuginosa • Rapid hair growth (cheeks\nose) • Hair-removing cream

NOTES:

Facial fistulas that leak when drinking can be plugged with silicone impression material (eg otoform from P C Werth Ltd., London).

See also Radiotherapy, Sweating, Steroids.

SPINAL CORD COMPRESSION

Symptoms	• Back pain (90%) • Weakness (both legs) • "Funny feelings" in legs • "Tired legs" (on stairs) • Bilateral root pain (on coughing) • Difficulty passing urine (late) • Patient may progress through these stages in hours
Signs	• Thoracic bony tenderness • Brisk reflexes • Upgoing plantars • A sensory level (nipple=T4, umbilicus=T10) • Urinary retention (late) • Peri-anal numbness (late)
Emergency treatment	• 16mg dexamethasone – immediately (PO or IV) • Radiotherapy – same day
Radiotherapy	• Same day! • If no MRI available the level can be judged by level of pain, previous bone scans and sensory level • Slowly developing lesions respond best
MRI scan	• Definitive investigation • Must include whole spine, as compression can occur at several levels • Do RT, first then scan, if it avoids delay
Neuro-surgery (rarely)	**Considered if:** • Biopsy is needed (diagnosis uncertain) • Progressive weakness despite radiotherapy • Spinal collapse • Cervical cord lesion
Cord Compression with paralysed legs	• Steroids may improve sphincter function • RT pointless except to control bone pain
Cauda equina compression	• Damage to nerve roots below LI • Cord ends at L1 • eg pelvic tumour with infiltration of the lumbo-sacral plexus <u>flaccid</u> weakness\absent reflexes • Sciatic pain (often bilateral) • Urinary hesitancy\retention

Cauda equina compression (continued)	• Peri-anal numbness ("saddle anesthesia") • Treatment non-urgent and is the same as for cord compression, but radiotherapy is often disappointing.
Management of established paraplegia	• Explain and discuss options • Adapt to wheelchair living • Catheter • Bowel regulation • Pressure area care • Avoid contractures (physio) • Social adjustment, home adaptions (OT) • Treat depression • Psychological adjustment (counselling) • Sexual counselling

NOTES:

Spinal cord compression is a medical emergency because prompt treatment within 1–2 days can prevent paraplegia, which is a devastating complication. If the patient can still walk at the time of treatment, 70% retain their mobility. But once the diagnosis is obvious the results are poor – therefore refer if suspicious! Once paralysed few will walk again.

It occurs in about 5% of cancers (breast, lung and prostate and myeloma, most commonly).

The median survival is poor (2–4 months) BUT 15% will survive 1 year and 10% 2 years.

Preventive treatment with RT can be given to patients with known vertebral metastases. All patients with spinal metastases and their relatives AND their primary care team should be <u>warned</u> to report urgently if any weakness or "funny feelings" occur in both legs – patients often ignore it until too late.

MRI scan is the definitive investigation, and must include the whole spine because there are often multiple levels of compression.

Steroids should not be withheld except in the rare situation of cord compression in an undiagnosed patient in case it is due to lymphoma, because biopsies become uninterpretable.

If paraplegia is already established urgent referral for investigations or treatment may not be appropriate, but RT may still be needed to control back pain.

Radiotherapy is the main treatment and can be given without prior MRI scan if it would cause a delay. The treatment level can be judged by the level of pain and the results of previous bone scans. The sensory level is not a reliable guide to treatment, because there may be several levels of compression. MRI scan should still be performed later, in case other areas of compression also need treating.

Bowel regulation is the best way of managing faecal incontinence due to a weak anal sphincter. It means allowing constipation and giving enemas, sometimes with a stimulant laxative such as senna, 2–3 times a week.

SPIRITUAL DISTRESS

Recognise distress as being spiritual
- "I'm frightened of not existing"
- "I feel so alone"
- "Why me? Am I being punished?"
- "I had so much to do"

"Change gear"
- Spiritual distress cannot be 'controlled' like a symptom, but it can be acknowledged.
- In addition to being a professional expert you can also be a human companion, willing to simply 'be there' to listen and affirm.

Acknowledge the deeper lever
- Ask: "What has been the most difficult aspect of this illness for you?"
- Ask: "How are you coping in yourself, in your spirits?"
- Ask: "Do you ever wonder why this has happened to you?"
- Ask: "Has this illness changed the way you think about life?"

Distinguish religious from spiritual
- Ask: "Do you believe in a 'Higher Power'?"
- Ask: "Do you believe in an after life?"
- Ask: "Is your religion a support to you?"

Maintain religious support
- Inform their minister of religion
- Show interest – ask about any religious requirements (diet, rituals, prayers, time alone etc)
- Is there a rota for pastoral visiting\helping?
- People with religious convictions still need ordinary spiritual support as well.

Find out what normally lifts their spirits
- What normally gives this person enjoyment?
- Anything that lifts a person's spirits is spiritually uplifting, from a bright smile, a cup of hot tea, a walk in the countryside or a meal with friends.

Ask about their life story
- Spiritual distress is often biographical distress ("It wasn't meant to be like this").
- Many people have regrets and guilt. Listening to a bit of someone's life story can help them to feel accepted, understood and less isolated.
- We should not talk about death without first talking about life, the high points and low points.
- Ask: "has any possible good come out of your illness?"

Discuss realistic short-term goals
- Realistic short-term goals can reduce hopelessness and fear.
- Goals can be enjoyed in four ways: planning them, discussing them, doing them and remembering them.
- Diaries or scrapbooks can be very helpful, especially if there are young children in the family

> "*I am having a wonderful time fixing treasures for my children. There are diaries and tapes of stories told and oral history which a friend has agreed to type up for me*"
> *Clare Vaughan, when terminally ill.*

Affirm the person as unique and accepted
- Being treated respectfully and patiently is affirming, and reduces the sense of isolation.
- "You matter because you are you"

Reduce the sense of powerlessness
- Many patients are distressed by the loss of control over their lives
- Share all decision-making
- Some patients find planning their own funeral restores a sense of control and for some it is creative and enjoyable.

Ask about a will
- Ask "Have you ever made a will?"
- Patients are often relieved to discuss it
- It is easier to leave a life that is tidied up, and it makes things much easier for the family afterwards

NOTES:

> "Every disease has two diagnoses, a medical one and a spiritual one" – *Paul Tournier*

Serious illness can bring a sense of isolation and hopelessness but also later a fresh perspective and a re-assessment of values and of what is important in life.

Trying to rescue someone from their spiritual distress is to undervalue their experience. Avoid philosophy – what is needed is listening and empathy. We need to "be with" and to be a companion, to listen and to learn.

It is possible for patients to re-frame their spiritual distress if they are given opportunities to talk about it (see Emotional Distress):

Why me?	– Why not me? Some others are worse off
I'm so alone	– I'm part of the world
It's hopeless	– I will focus on one day at a time
I'm frightened	– I've seen some people die peacefully
My life is a mess	– Some good things have happened

STEROIDS

What problems can be helped by steroids?	• Anorexia • Dyspnoea due to lymphangitis • Malignant dysphagia • Pyloric obstruction • SVC compression • Nerve pain • Intractable nausea • Cord compression • Brain metastases
How do they work?	• Mechanism is unknown • Presumed to reduce peri-tumour oedema
What dose of dexamethasone?	• 2–4mg daily for anorexia • 8–16mg daily for high-dose trial • Stop after 5 days if not helping.
What dose for brain metastases?	• 16mg dexamethasone daily • Reduces peri-tumour oedema • Increase to 32mg may have a place • 80% improve for 1–2 months
What route?	• Oral as effective as IV\SC, after 24 hours • IV for emergencies (SVCO or cord compression). • SC infusion for dysphagia or vomiting
What are equivalent doses of different steroids?	• Hydrocortisone 30mg • Prednisolone 7mg • Dexamethasone 1mg
Do replacement steroids need to be continued?	• Yes, because dexamethasone and prednisolone do not have sufficient mineralocorticoid activity. • Replacement steroids are cortisone acetate 20mg BD or hydrocortisone 20mg and fludrocortisone 0.1mg daily.
What should the patient be told?	• Take early (to avoid insomnia) • Don't stop suddenly • Side-effects are common • Improvement does not mean tumour regression. • Carry steroid card

What are the common side-effects?	• Oral thrush (40%) • Facial swelling (30%) • Oedema (20%) • Dyspepsia (5%) • Diabetes (5%) • Weight gain (4%) • Insomnia (3%)
What are the effects on the skin?	• Thinning of skin • Purpura • Easy bruising • Facial hair growth • Striae (purple stretch marks) • Reduce dose if possible
What about Peptic Ulceration?	• Increased incidence of peptic ulcer is probably due to concurrent NSAIDS • Add PPI to cover steroids plus NSAID • Avoid if active ulceration
What if the patient is diabetic?	• Blood glucose rises. • Benefits may still outweigh the inconvenience of worsened diabetes. • A patient on hypogycaemics may need to start insulin. Insulin needs increase – monitor.
How are steroids stopped?	• If given for less than 1 week steroids can be stopped immediately • Otherwise reduce gradually down to 0.5mg prednisolone alternate days for 1 week before stopping (to avoid adrenal crisis and hypotension).

NOTES:

40% of hospice patients benefit from steroids for a variety of symptoms, but the useful effect can wear off after a few weeks and side-effects can be very troublesome. Therefore the aim is to achieve the lowest dose that controls the symptom. Review regularly and reduce the dose if possible.

STOMA CARE

Types of Stoma:	• End Colostomy (permanent, defunctioning) • Loop Colostomy (temporary, decompressing) • End ileostomy • Loop ileostomy (prior to ileo-anal pouch) • Urostomy (following ileal conduit or ureterostomy)
Types of Appliance (one piece, or two piece + flange)	• Closed pouch • Drainable (post-op) • Urostomy (tap and valve) • Fistula (large, drainable)
Stoma accessories	• Pastes to fill crevices (eg Comfeel) • Powders to protect skin (eg Orahesive) • Protective skin films (eg Derma-gard) • Barrier creams to prevent itching (eg Comfeel) • Deodorants (eg Atmocol, Ostobon) • Belts (to secure pouch) • Pouch covers (to reduce sweating) • Clips (to close drainable bags) • Stoma corsets (for parastomal hernias). • Specialist clothing (underwear, swimwear)
Skin soreness	• Frequent change of appliance (? leakage) • Excoriation • Eczeme\Allergy • Bacterial infection (rare) • Fungal infection (mostly with urostomy)
What can be done about leakage	• Ill-fitting appliance? (may be due to weight loss) • Wafers, powders, pastes • Convex insets/appliances • Re-site
What is irrigation?	• Wash-outs every 1–3 days • Irrigation sets needed • 500–1200cc water instilled • Takes 30–60 minutes • Patient doesn't wear a bag, but usually wears a stoma cap, mini-pouch or conseal plug which incorporate a charcoal filter. • Not recommended for palliative surgery

How is diarrhoea managed?	• Codeine phosphate 30–60mg QID or • Loperamide 2–4mg QID • Daily bulking agent eg Fybogel
How is Constipation managed?	• Increase fluids • Decrease nuts, eggs, rice • Oral laxatives • Microlette or arachis oil enemas can be given via a colostomy if necessary • Glycerine suppositories are not effective
What surgical problems occur?	• Prolapse • Para-stomal hernia • Stenosis • Obstruction • Bleeding (Cryo?) • Perforation (BLACK MUCOSA = ISCHAEMIA)
What problems can be diet-related?	• Flatus (onions, pulses, green veg) • Odour (eggs, cheese, fish) • Diarrhoea (salad, fruit, spices) • Blockage (high fibre foods)
Can suppositories be used?	• Suppositories are not always retained • by a stoma, but a diazepam enema (Stesolid) is usually effective via a stoma.

NOTES:

A stoma is a surgically created opening of the bowel (or urinary tract) on to the body surface.

Stomas are managed either with an appliance or with irrigation (when the bowel is washed out twice a day, so no bag is needed). Irrigation may be useful short-term to heal very excoriated skin.

Modern closed pouches incorporate a skin-protective barrier and a charcoal filter.

SUBCUTANEOUS INFUSIONS 1 – Drugs

DRUG	24 HOUR DOSE	NOTES
Diamorphine (5, 10, 30, 100, 500mg)	5–1000mg	• Opioid of choice for SC infusions • Highly soluble • Dose=one third of 24h morphine dose • Compatible with ALL drugs below
Cyclizine (50mg in 1ml)	100–150mg	• Must be diluted with water for injection (not saline). • Precipitates above 25mg\ml. • Can logically be combined with haloperidol for difficult nausea or vomiting. Often causes skin irritation. • Not compatible with: high dose diamorphine (above 25mg\ml), metoclopramide, dexamethasone or octreotide.
Haloperidol (5mg in 1ml)	5–20mg	• May precipitate above 1mg\ml • Mixes well with all other drugs • Used as an anti-emetic at lower dose, or for sedation if agitated or paranoid at higher dose, eg 10–20mg.
Metoclopramide* (10mg in 2ml)	40–100mg	• Takes up a large volume, eg 80mg is 16ml of fluid, so high doses need a large or separate syringe. • Will not mix with ondansetron • Risk of dystonic reaction in higher doses.
Levomepromazine (25mg in 1ml)	6.25–12.5mg	• Can also be given as a single SC injection daily as it is long-acting. • It is also used in higher doses 25–200mg as a powerful sedative for terminal agitation • Will not mix with dexamethasone or octreotide.
Midazolam* (10mg in 2ml)	10–120mg	• Anxiolytic (in low dose) or sedative (in higher dose) with a retrograde amnesic effect. • Useful for terminal agitation. • It will not mix with dexamethasone.

*these drugs take up a large volume in higher doses

DRUG	24 HOUR DOSE	NOTES
Dexamethasone (8mg in 2ml)	4–16mg	• Consider giving as a single daily IM injection, as it is long-acting. • Will not mix with cyclizine, levomepromazine, glycopyronium or midazolam.
Hyoscine hydrobromide (0.4mg in 1ml)	1.2–2.4mg	• For terminal bubbling ("death rattle"). • Mixes well with other drugs
Hyoscine butylbromide (Buscopan) (20mg in 1ml)	60–120mg	• For colic. • Mixes well with other drugs
Glycopyronium (200mcg in 1 ml)	1.2mg	• Dries respiratory secretions. • Causes less tachycardia or drowsiness than hyoscine, and is cheaper. • Precipitates with dexamethasone.
Octreotide (100mcg in 1ml) (500mcg in 1ml)	300–900mcg	• Reduces gastro-intestinal secretions (in vomiting or diarrhoea or from fistulas) and reduces gut motility (colic). • Does not mix with cyclizine, dexamethasone or levomepromazine. • If using longterm consider single injection of long-acting lanreotide.
Ondansetron (4mg in 2ml)	16–24mg	• Versatile broad-spectrum anti-emetic. • Will not mix with metoclopramide
Ketorolac (30mg in 1ml)	60–90mg	• Useful for severe bone pain. • Mixes poorly with most other drugs (because it is alkaline and most of the other drugs are acidic). • Use a separate syringe and pump.
Hyaluronidase (1500i.u. per amp)	1500i.u.	• Increases diffusion of fluids through subcutaneous tissues. • Compatible with other drugs in infusions, but probably better to inject SC straight into the site where the infusion needle will go.

Indications for use
- Persistent nausea and vomiting
- Dysphagia
- Intestinal obstruction
- Too weak to swallow medication (e.g. dying)
- Sleepiness / coma
- Poor alimentary absorption (rare)
- If parenteral drugs are more effective (rare)

Prepare the patient and family
- Demonstrate the pump
- Explain the procedure
- Discuss site for the needle
- Invite questions
- Acknowledge anxieties and reassure
- Provide written instructions

Equipment needed:
- Syringe driver + hard plastic cover
- Key rate adjuster or paper clip
- 9–volt alkaline battery × 2 (the patient is given a spare)
- 20ml Luer lock syringe (or 30ml)
- Butterfly needle with 100cm line (FSB034)
- Transparent film dressing, e.g. Tegaderm, Opsite
- Drugs +Water for injection
- Sticky label for syringe (drug doses)
- Holster
- Syringe driver chart

The Graseby MS26 (Green)

MS26 can fit 2,5,10,20,30, and 35 ml syringes of various brands

Syringes only fit the pump if underfilled

        10ml syringe = 9.5mls
        20ml syringe = 16mls
        30ml syringe = 21mls

- 24 hourly device (mm per 24 hour)
- Small (16 × 5 × 2 cm)
- Light (185 g) and portable
- 9V battery lasts for 54 deliveries
- 0–60 mm scale (to measure fluid length)
- Boost button (DO NOT USE)
- Flashing light (once every 25 seconds)
- Alarm (sounds for 15 seconds if infusion blocks)
- Dial 0–60mm per 24 hr
- There is no off switch (remove battery)

The Graseby MS16A (Blue)
- Hourly device (1–99 mm per hour)
- Generally used for 12 hour infusions (or shorter)
- 48 mm of fluid set at 4 mm per hour lasts 12 hours

Common sites for needle
- Upper arms (not in bedbound)
- Chest wall/abdominal wall
- Anterior thigh
- Upper back (useful if restless)

Setting it up
- Check equipment and draw up drugs
- Prime the cannula first (0.75ml), then
- Measure the length of the fluid in the syringe (ruler on pump)
- Do not include the width of the rubber bung in the syringe
- Set rate on counter using the red adjusting key or a paper clip (NOT point of scissors)
- EG fluid length 50 mm, set dial to 50 mm per 24 hours
- Contents of the syringe will then be infused over 24 hours
- Check 4 hourly (site, no leaks, rate, volume remaining, no precipitate, light still flashing)

SYRINGE DRIVER – PROBLEMS	
Won't start	• batteries – right way?
Stops flashing	• Low battery – will still run for 24h
Infusion too slow (ie volume remaining more than expected)	• Tube disconnected? • Tube kinked? • Syringe displaced? • Inflamed site? • Blocked needle?
Infusion too fast	• Check rate setting
Precipitate of drugs	• Discard mixture • Increase dilution • Use 30ml syringe?+ • Simplify regime? • Use 2 pumps? • (NB. Change syringe and line and re-site)

NOTES:
The Graseby MS26 (Green) is the syringe driver recommended for palliative care. Insert battery (alarm sounds to show battery is OK). Press and hold down start button. Once alarm stops, release button – this STARTS pump. Motor whirrs for a few seconds only, then every 3 minutes. If the light stops flashing the pump will still continue to operate for the remainder of that syringe.

SURGERY (palliative)

Debulking of tumour	• Enhances effect of RT or CT
Laser	• Debulking (eg rectum) • Re-canalizing (eg oesophagus, bronchus, trachea) • Control of bleeding
Excision of Metastases	• lung, liver or brain • Usually for solitary metastases when local disease is controlled and there is no evidence of other metastases.
Palliative colostomy	• For malignant intestinal obstruction when resection and anastomosis is not possible
Local control of Tumour	• For discharge or bleeding • To reduce disfigurement • Debridement • Skin graft may be indicated
P-V shunt	• Can control ascites for several months
Oesophageal tube	• For unresectable tumours or fistulas • RT can be given before or after • 90% get good swallowing
Stents	• Biliary stent for jaundice • Ureteric stent for colic • Tracheal stent for stridor • SVC stent for SVC obstruction
Urinary procedures	• Ileal conduit • Nephrostomy • Ureteric stent • Ureteric implant
Fixation of fractures	• Internal fixation whenever possible, which allows easier nursing even if mobility is not restored (see Fractures).
Gastrostomy	• PEG is preferred to open gastrostomy • Indicated for dysphagia causing hunger or thirst in a patient with weeks to live

Tracheostomy	• For stridor and dyspnoea due to laryngeal damage
Pleural surgery	• For recurrent effusions • Pleuradesis • Pleurectomy
Pericardial surgery	• For recurrent effusion • Balloon pericardiotomy is effective and safer than a pericardial window at open surgery
Neurosurgery	• Solitary brain metastasis • Laminectomy for cord compression • Cordotomy for pain • Implanted spinal cord stimulation • Hypophysectomy (rarely)
Amputation	• Last resort • Non-functioning limb • Control of tumour not possible

NOTES:

Discuss options with the patient very carefully. It can be very difficult for a patient with far-advanced disease to contemplate the idea of having surgery.

There is a high risk of thrombosis in advanced cancer. Patients having abdominal or orthopaedic surgery should have prophylactic anticoagulation with dalteparin (2500 units 2 hours pre-operatively then daily until mobile. 5000 units if high risk).

Excellent communication between patient and family, palliative care team and surgeons is needed.

SVC COMPRESSION

Features of SVC compression	• Not life-threatening, but distressing • Headaches (worse after bending over) • Blurred vision • Dizziness\fainting • Siezures • Facial swelling • Swollen eyes\neck\arms (tight collar and rings) • Hoarse voice (recurrent laryngeal nerve) • Pink eyes • Peri-orbital oedema • Dilated neck veins (non-pulsatile) • Dilated collateral veins (chest, arms) • Stridor\dyspnoea due to tracheal oedema (late) • Pleural effusion (late) • Pericardial effusion (late)
SVC Stent	• For severe symptoms • 90% get rapid relief
Radiotherapy	• Relieves symptoms • Steroid cover prevents initial swelling and worsening of symptoms • 20 Gy in 5 fractions (80% improve within 3–14 days)
Chemotherapy (may be preferred to RT)	• Small-cell lung • Lymphoma • Testicular cancer
Steroids	• Dexamethasone 8–12mg\day • Can produce a second remission
Emergency Treatment if severe	• 100% oxygen • IV dexamethasone 20mg • IV frusemide 40–80mg

NOTES:

SVC compression is usually due to lung cancer (80%). If a patient presents with SVC compression it is essential to get histology as treatment depends on tumour type. Although described as a radiotherapy emergency there is usually time to investigate and plan treatment. Emergency measures are only needed for very late presentation with severe symptoms. Scans may reveal SVC thrombosis rather than compression – treated with thrombolysis.

Reversible Cause?	• Infection? (MSU, swabs, blood cultures) • Thyrotoxicosis • Hypoglycaemia • Drug-induced? (tamoxifen, megestrol, bleomycin, LHRH analogues (eg goserelin), pilocarpine, co-proxamol or morphine, in some patients)
Hot flushes?	• Can occur in men (castration, anti-androgens) • Consider Hormone replacement
Paracetamol or NSAID	• Effective for neoplastic fever
Anti-cholinergic drugs	• Often tried because sweating is mediated by acetyl choline • Often unsuccessful.
Consider changing opioid	• If morphine is suspected • Change to fentanyl or oxycodone
Thalidomide	• Can be very effective • Drowsiness, nausea (can be severe) • May block tumour-induced cytokines • Handle with care (very dangerous to pregnant women)
Nursing care	• Encourage fluids • Use cotton linen • Regular changes of bedclothes • Use a fan • Sponging

NOTES:

Normal sweating is part of the temperature control mechanism of the body, cooling the body by evaporation. The normal volume of sweat produced is about 500ml per day, but can rise to as high as 2 litres per hour in severe sweating. Sweat glands (eccrine glands) are found over the whole body and are stimulated by acetyl choline. But the sweat glands on the palms and soles are different – they are only stimulated by adrenaline in response to embarrassment or fear.

Sweating in advanced cancer is a para-neoplastic phenomenon, and is more common in lymphomas and in tumours with liver metastases, but can occur with any advanced malignancy. It can occur with or without fever. It is probably due to chemical factors released by the tumour and acting on the temperature contol centre in the hypothalamus.

Regular changes of bed linen is all that can be offered some patients. Ensure that the laundry facilities are adequate.

TERMINAL PHASE

Nursing care	<ul><li>2 hourly mouth care</li><li>2 hourly turning</li><li>Ripple mattress</li><li>Catheterize?</li><li>Counselling</li></ul>
Mouth care	<ul><li>Frequent sips (beaker)</li><li>Moisten mouth regularly with foamstick (relatives can do this)</li><li>Crushed ice to suck</li><li>Vaseline on lips</li></ul>
Dry eyes	<ul><li>Hypromellose eye drops</li></ul>
Pressure sores	<ul><li>Zinc and castor oil ointment under a dry dressing reduces friction (comfort is the priority at this stage)</li><li>NSAID for pain</li></ul>
Agitation	<ul><li>Full bladder?</li><li>Pain?</li><li>Sedate (see notes)</li></ul>
SC infusion of drugs	<ul><li>Useful when unable to swallow</li><li>A common combination is – Diamorphine (50% oral dose) – Levomepromazine 50–100mg\24h – Hyoscine 0.8–2.4mg\24h</li></ul>
Pain on movement	<ul><li>Indomethacin suppositories 100mg BD</li></ul>
Dyspnoea	<ul><li>100% oxygen</li><li>Midazolam with diamorphine</li></ul>
Twitching Myoclonic jerks	<ul><li>Midazolam 20–90mg\24hrs SC</li><li>Rectal diazepam (Stesolid) 10–40mg PRN</li><li>Phenobarbitone 400–800\24hrs SC</li></ul>
Picking at sheets	<ul><li>Due to hallucinations</li><li>Haloperidol 5–10mg\24h SC</li></ul>
Regurgitation	<ul><li>Nasogastric aspiration</li></ul>
Bubbling	<ul><li>"Death rattle"</li><li>Re-position patient</li><li>Hyoscine 0.2–0.4mg 4 hourly</li><li>Glycopyronium 0.2mg 6 hourly</li><li>Frusemide 40mg IM or IV</li><li>Scopaderm patch (hyoscine 0.5mg released over 72 hours)</li><li>Suction (with a soft catheter)</li></ul>

Dehydration	• Ice chips to suck • 2 hourly mouth care • Thirst is rare • Explain to family if necessary that IV fluids do not increase comfort.
Thirst (rare)	• IV fluids • S.C. fluids can be infused at 50–100ml\hour (i.e. 1.2 – 2.4 L\day). The thigh (or both thighs) is the best sight. Hyalase is not necessary • Tap water enema (?)
Bleeding	• Reverse warfarin with vitamin K • Midazolam if patient distressed
Family support	• Explain all proceedures • Explain changes of dying • Offer to meet family together • Rota for visiting?
Religious requirements	• The important rule is to discuss religious needs with the patient and family, and avoid making assumptions.
After death	• Prayers at the bedside • Last offices • Tubes and catheters are removed • Wounds covered with adhesive dressing to prevent leakage • Pacemaker removed

NOTES:

The Terminal phase is characterized by day-to-day deterioration. The common symptoms in the terminal 48 hours are listed on page 7.

A peaceful death is important for the relatives as well as the patient: "*How people die remains in the memory of those who live on*" (Cicely Saunders). Families often find it comforting if carers continue to talk to the patient even after unconsciousness eg "I am just going to touch your eyelash to see how sleepy you are".

Sedation for terminal agitation or distress should be prompt. It can be allowed to wear off once the patient is settled and any reversible causes have been treated, to see if sedation is still necessary. Long term sedation (rarely needed) raises the ethical dilemma of intravenous fluids (see Ethical Problems).

THROMBOSIS

Assessment	• Unilateral leg swelling • Pain • Chest pain\dyspnoea (PEs)? • Tenderness (behind knee\anterior thigh) • Oedema • Cyanosis of the leg (late) • Dilated superficial veins (late). • Positive venogram\ultrasound
Analgesia	• Anti-coagulation reduces pain • Morphine often needed initially
Elastic support stocking	• Thigh-length • Remove at night • Adequate treatment for a below-knee DVT

Anti-coagulation	• Indicated for
	  • pain
	  • severe swelling
	  • DVT in thigh (PE more likely)
	  • PEs

IVC filter	• An option for a relatively fit patient if anti-coagulation is not preventing PE's or if it is risky, eg active bleeding or vascular brain metastases (renal, melanoma) • Additional anti-coagulation may still be needed for leg symptoms
Dalteparin (Fragmin)	• Treatment of choice for thrombosis • Single daily SC injection • Onset 2 hours, duration 10–24 hours • 12,500u to treat DVT (200u per kg) • 18,000u is maximum dose • Single dose syringes of 2500, 5000, 10000, 12500, 15000, 18000 units • Given for around 5 days (till warfarin is stabilized by INR) • Monitoring not needed • Partially reversed by protamine (if bleeding occurs) • Other LMWHs are certoparin (Alphaparin), enoxaparin (Clexane) and tinazparin (Innohep).

Warfarin	• Loading dose (10mg day 1, 10mg day 2)
	• Give at same time (evening) each day
	• Check INR daily (morning) from day 4
	• Normal dose range = 3–9mg daily.
	• Given for 6–12 weeks
	• 5% risk of major haemorrhage
INR	• Daily INR for first few days, then every 1–2 weeks
	• Aim· 2–3 for DVT\PE
	3–4.5 if recurrent
	• Above 4.5 – omit warfarin for 2 days
	• Above 7 consider Vitamin K, 0.5mg IV
	• Recurrent thrombosis occurs in 15% despite therapeutic INR

NOTES:

Thrombosis is much more common in cancer (probably cytokines activating coagulation). 15% of cancer patients get symptoms of thrombosis, but 50% have thrombosis at post mortem! Patients at high risk are those having surgery or IV chemotherapy or those with indwelling catheters.

Anti-coagulation is indicated for severe pain or swelling or for recurrent pulmonary emboli. Below knee DVT can often be managed with an elastic support stocking and analgesia.

Warfarin is potentiated by: dextropropoxyphene, NSAIDs, quinidine, omeprazole, tamoxifen, flutamide, ketoconazole, fluconazole, metronidazole, co-trimoxazole, chloramphenicol, ciprofloxacin, and ifosphamide.

NB Warfarin can be reversed with vitamin K, 2–5mg, slowly IV.

Swelling of the ARM may be due to:

– lymphoedema	– unilateral
– SVCO	– bilateral
– Axillary vein thrombosis	– unilateral

IVC thrombosis causes swelling of both legs.

URINARY PROBLEMS

Frequency	<ul><li>Disimpact faeces</li><li>Reduce diuretics</li><li>MSU <u>then</u> antibiotics</li></ul>
Nocturnal Frequency	<ul><li>Exclude infection\impaction</li><li>Frusemide 20–40mg mane</li><li>Imipramine 10–50mg nocte</li><li>Urinary sheath\pouch</li><li>Desmopressin 100–300mcg nocte</li></ul>
Urgency	<ul><li>Exclude infection\impaction</li><li>Imipramine 10–50mg nocte</li><li>Oxybutinin 5mg TID</li></ul>
Incontinence	<ul><li>Exclude infection\impaction</li><li>Urinary sheath</li><li>Penis pouch</li><li>Disposable underpads</li><li>Catheter</li><li>Vaginal prosthesis</li><li>Ileal conduit\ureteric implant</li><li>Refer to incontinence adviser or consultant urologist?</li></ul>
Stress incontinence	<ul><li>Vaginal ring pessary – 74mm</li><li>Dienoestrol Cream</li><li>Oestradiol lmg daily</li></ul>
Large volume of urine	<ul><li>Treat diabetes\hypercalcaemia,</li><li>Diabetes insipidus</li><li>Anxiety and over-drinking?</li><li>Desmopressin (see notes)</li></ul>
Vesico-vaginal fistula	<ul><li>Dribbling incontinence</li><li>Surgical diversion (ileal conduit or uretero-sigmoidostomy)</li><li>Vaginal prosthesis</li><li>Hygiene ++</li><li>Desmopressin (see notes)</li></ul>
Retention	<ul><li>Spinal cord compression?</li><li>Disimpact loaded rectum</li><li>Stop anticholinergics</li><li>Catheter</li><li>Suprapubic catheter (stricture)</li><li>Alpha-blocking drug</li><li>TURP or repeat TURP</li></ul>
Coloured urine	<ul><li>Blood</li><li>Bile due to jaundice</li><li>Dark urine due to dehyration</li><li>Danthron from laxatives</li><li>Rifampicin</li><li>Beetroot\food additives</li></ul>

CATHETERS		
Indications for a catheter	<ul><li>Prevention of pressure sores</li><li>Pain on moving</li><li>Weakness</li><li>Incontinence</li><li>Retention</li><li>Need for physical comfort</li></ul>	
Catheter care	<ul><li>Sterile insertion</li><li>5–10ml balloon</li><li>14–22G</li><li>No routine changing</li><li>No routine irrigation</li><li>No antibiotics for asymptomatic bacteriuria</li><li>Irrigate only for blockage</li><li>Leakage <u>more</u> likely with bigger size due to loss of urethral tone</li></ul>	
Catheter problems	<ul><li>Infection</li><li>Bladder spasms</li><li>Urethritis</li><li>Blocking</li><li>Encrustation</li></ul>	– CSU then antibiotics – Antispasmodics – Swab, lignocaine gel – Irrigate – Change catheter if spasms occuring
Clots	<ul><li>Citrate bladder washout</li><li>Irrigate with 3–way catheter</li><li>Haematuria catheter</li><li>Cystoscopic removal</li><li>Avoid tranexamic acid</li></ul>	
Bladder washouts	<ul><li>Indicated for debris (to prevent blocks)</li><li>Sodium chloride (solution S) is as effective as chlorhexidine (C) or the more complex solutions (G or R).</li><li>Use sodium citrate solution to dissolve clots</li></ul>	

NOTES:

Desmopressin (100mcg tablets) inhibits the renal production of urine, and a dose of 100–200mcg at night can be useful if nocturnal frequency is disturbing sleep.

Oxybutinin (Ditropan) 5mg TID reduces bladder spasms, urgency or strangury.

Alpha blockers eg indoramin (Baratol, Doralese) 20mg BD relax the smooth muscle of the urethra and can relieve benign prostatic symptoms in patients unable to have a TURP, but they tend to cause hypotension.

Incontinence sheaths (Uridom) for male patients avoid the need to insert a catheter. Self-adhesive. 4 sizes.

Penis pouches (Hollister) are used if the penis is retracted and a sheath cannot be fitted. It fits like a colostomy bag over the penis.

WEAKNESS

Exclude Reversible Causes	• Anaemia • Depression • Infection • Parkinson's • Drugs (Hypotensives, Baclofen, steroids, diuretics)
Steroids	• Dexamethasone 2–4mg daily • Improves well-being more than physical strength • Risk of proximal myopathy
Blood transfusion	• Weakness is often due to disease • progression more than anaemia • Short-lived effect (but may be worthwhile eg for a special occasion)
Physiotherapy	• Maintains strength • Optimizes mobility • Teach relatives (lifting, transferring) • Walking aids
Wheelchair	• Involve OT in selection • Can increase independence • Occasional use (eg shopping) or • Permanent use <u>with</u> cushion
Splints	• Useful for nerve palsies causing localized weakness (eg wrist drop, foot drop)
Occupational Therapy	• Adjust daily living • Home assessment • Household adaptions • Address issue of boredom • Reminiscence work
Explanation	• Part of illness • Strength fluctuates • No specific antidote • Periods of rest may need to be prescribed
Rota for Visitors	• Patient may need protecting from excessive visiting
Counselling	• Allow patient to express emotions (frustration, anger and sadness) • Adjustment to limitations is both physical and psychological

NOTES:

Anaemia (Hb below 8g\dl) in advanced cancer is usually normocytic anaemia (with MCV in the normal range of 76-96 fl) due to chronic disease, and is usually treated with blood transfusion if it is causing symptoms (provided the patient is not actively bleeding, since transfusion just worsens the bleeding). If platelets are also low (below $100 \times 10^9/L$) it suggests marrow infiltration, which has a poor prognosis. Oral iron is given if the anaemia is microcytic (MCV below 76 fl) suggesting iron deficiency due to chronic blood loss, and should increase the Hb by about 1g per week provided the marrow is normal. *Epoetin* (Eprex, Recormon) usually just called "Epo" is genetically engineered human erythropoetin, a hormone produced by the kidney that stimulates the bone marrow to produce red blood cells. A weekly injection (which is painful) can increase Hb by 1g per month. A usual dose is 25,000 units for a 60kg man (450u per kg). If response is poor the dose can be doubled. The main side-effect is hypertension. Patients with marrow failure do not respond and iron supplements should also be given (because a low iron will prevent a response). Some manufactures offer special support such as a nurse to visit the patient. It is very expensive.

Localized weakness may be due to brain metastases, CVA (sudden onset), cord compression (both legs), malignant nerve damage (painful), peripheral neuropathy (foot drop), steroid myopathy (hip weakness) or nerve palsies.

Physiotherapy is beneficial for 50% of hospice patients. Exercise seems the natural antidote to weakness, and it is often possible to improve mobility and independence.

Occupational Therapy can be invaluable in helping the patient adjust to weakness, make adaptions to their home and lifestyle, and in overcoming the problem of boredom.

Boredom is a common problem. Company, outings, entertainments, creative activities, alteration of routines, TV, tapes and reminiscence (biography therapy) can all help.

Visitors can be a dilemma for some weak patients. The support is welcome, but too many visitors can be very exhausting. Discuss the patient's wishes. What is supportive? What is exhausting? A medical edict can help ("the doctor says"). Consider a rota for visitors.

Carcinomatous peripheral neuropathy (foot drop, numbness, burning pain) occurs in 2% of patients.

Rare causes of weakness are ectopic ACTH (treatable with metyrapone) or the Lambert-Eaton syndrome both seen in small cell (oat cell) lung cancer.

WEIGHT LOSS

Explanation	• Weight loss is related to cancer • Metabolism is altered, with an increased metabolic rate, plus marked muscle wasting due to a proteolysis-inducing factor. • Not reversed by high-calorie intake
Skin Care	• Pressure sores can occur over bony prominences (hip, spine) • Educate and prevent
Photographs	• Can help adjust to an altered body shape • Old photographs show carers how the patient still thinks of themselves. • New family photographs can demonstrate that a person is still part of the family circle.
New clothes	• clothes that fit can be a great boost to morale.
Dentist	• Loose dentures can be relined at the bedside. This improves chewing and facial appearance and lasts several months.
Optician	• Loose spectacles can be adjusted to fit.
Physiotherapy	• improves mobility (walking\transferring) • iimproves morale.
Spiritual support	• The real fear may be dying rather than weight loss ("I'm wasting away, soon there will be nothing left").

NOTES:

Cachexia is a para-neoplastic phenomenon consisting of marked weight loss, weakness and anorexia. It occurs in up to 50% of patients with advanced cancer. It may partly be due to cytokines produced by the tumour (or in response to the tumour) such as tumour necrosis factor, interleukin-6 and interleukin-1. Ibuprofen may possibly reduce this cytokine effect in some patients.

NB Avoid routine weighing which becomes demoralizing.

WOUND HEALING

PHASES OF WOUND HEALING

PHASE	TIME	PROCESS
1 Vascular	MINUTES	• Vasoconstriction, clotting, platelet plug
2. Inflammatory	DAYS (2–3)	• Exudate, leucocytes, macrophages
3. Granulation tissue forms (pink)	WEEKS (1–2)	• Fibroblasts lay down collagen and "ground substance" • New capilliaries grow in • Re-epithelialization, new skin grows over the top from edges • Scab on top of new skin detaches
4. Scar maturation (white)	MONTHS	• Pink ground substance re-modelled into white avascular connective tissue scar. • If process goes wrong keloid can form.

DRESSINGS

- **Low adherence** (eg paraffin gauze, Tulle Gras, Release)
- **Semi-permeable** film (Bioclusive, Opsite, Tegaderm)
  - "Extra layer of skin" to prevent ulceration
  - Waterproof but allows oxygen in
  - Fall off if there is exudate
- **Hydrocolloid** (eg Comfeel, Granuflex)
  - Maintain hydration and temperature
  - Promote granulation tissue
  - Last a week
- **Hydrogel** (eg Intrasite, Hydrosorb)
  - Moisten slough
  - Need to be covered with film to keep moist
- **Alginate** (eg Kaltostat, Sorbsan)
  - Absorbent and haemostatic
- **Foam** (eg Lyafoam)
  - Absorbs exudate
- **Odour-absorbent** (eg Artisorb, Carbonet)
  - Reduce smell
  - Contain activated charcoal
  - Placed on top of other dressings

Larval therapy	
	• Removes slough
	• Explain carefully – some patients refuse
	• Well described by Pare (1579), Larry (1832), Zaccharias (1904)
	• Sterile maggots of greenbottle fly used (Lucilia sericata)
	• Available from Biosurgical Research Unit, Brigend
	• Liquefy dead tissue (with enzymes) then feed on it
	• Harmless to normal skin or tissue
	• Available in a muslin bag to lay on wound
	• Wound gets more pink and exudative with characteristic odour
	• Larvae grow from 2mm to 10mm over 2–3 days
	• Larvae do not hatch into flies for another 9 days
	• Importance may increase due to antibiotic resistance
Nutrition	
	• Protein is necessary for wound healing
	• Albumin >30g\L may not be possible in advanced disease
	• Hb ideally above 10g\dL
	• Vitamin C 500mg daily if malnourished
	• Zinc only necessary if deficient

NOTES:

Wound healing is delayed by malignant cells, movement or mechanical stress, foreign bodies, toxic cleansing agents and cold fluids.

Dressings are designed to promote moist wound healing, and avoid the need for frequent changes.

Ultrasound therapy may promote granulation tissue, but light does not.

Pseudomonas aeruginosa commonly colonizes chronic ulcers and will delay wound healing because it produces proteoses that damage the tissues. It rarely invades the tissues and antibiotics are rarely indicated. Alginate dressings improve healing.

Growth factors (cytokines) control the chronological process of wound healing. Growth factor therapy may become available to promote wound healing.

INDEX + ABBREVIATIONS

162

INDEX + ABBREVIATIONS

INDEX + ABBREVIATIONS

INDEX + ABBREVIATIONS

INDEX + ABBREVIATIONS